THE KIDNEY-FRIENDLY FOOD LIST

A Renal Diet Reference for Everyday Cooking

Nourish Your Health with Comprehensive Food List and Reliable Guidance

By RenalTracker Publishing

TABLE OF CONTENTS

Introduction

About This Book

Purpose and Scope

Navigating the complexities of kidney disease can feel overwhelming, especially when it comes to managing your diet. This book is designed to provide clear, comprehensive guidance to help you make informed nutritional decisions at every stage of chronic kidney disease (CKD). Our goal is to present dietary recommendations that are both evidence-based and practical for everyday life.

The food items featured in this guide have been carefully selected using trusted food databases and reputable scientific sources. Each recommendation reflects current nutritional research and established clinical guidelines to support optimal kidney health.

How to Use This Book

This guide is intended for anyone seeking to manage kidney disease through diet, whether you are newly diagnosed or looking for ways to refine your current approach. The content is organized for easy reference, allowing you to quickly find the information most relevant to your needs. Whether you are looking for foods to prioritize or limit, meal planning strategies, or kidney-friendly recipes, you will find structured guidance throughout these pages.

Foods are categorized to help you quickly identify options appropriate for kidney health. The comprehensive food lists are grounded in scientific research and crafted by our dedicated team of dietitians and nephrology nurses, providing a highly reliable foundation for your dietary decisions.

In addition to the food lists, you will find practical meal plans and recipes tailored to different stages of CKD. These tools are designed to help you maintain balance, variety, and nutritional adequacy while managing dietary restrictions.

For quick reference, use the detailed index on page 170 to locate specific foods or topics, and consult the glossary for clarification of key terms. Additional resources are included to further support your journey.

Managing kidney disease is an ongoing process. With the right knowledge and structured guidance, you can approach it with clarity and confidence.

Chapter 1: Understanding Chronic Kidney Disease

In my previous book, *Avoid Dialysis Diet Plan for Kidney Disease*, I extensively discussed the crucial role of diet in both the progression and management of kidney disease. However, before diving into the specifics of this guide, let's take a moment to recap what we're dealing with, how we reached this point, and the primary reason you are reading this book. (If you feel confident in your understanding of CKD basics, you are welcome to skip ahead to the next chapter!)

So, What is Kidney Disease?

Kidney disease occurs when the kidneys become damaged and can no longer filter blood effectively. This damage can lead to the accumulation of waste products in the body and may trigger other health complications that jeopardize your overall well-being.

For many individuals, kidney damage develops gradually over several years, often as a result of diabetes or high blood pressure. This condition is known as chronic kidney disease (CKD). Conversely, when kidney function declines suddenly due to illness, injury, or certain medications, it is referred to as acute kidney injury. This condition can affect individuals with previously normal kidney function or those with existing kidney issues, and it may be reversible.

The Growing Concern of Kidney Disease

Kidney disease is an escalating public health concern. More than 37 million Americans may be living with kidney disease, and countless others are at risk. Anyone, regardless of age or ethnicity, can develop kidney disease. The primary risk factors include:

- Diabetes

- High blood pressure

- Cardiovascular disease (affecting the heart and blood vessels)
- A family history of kidney failure
- Unhealthy lifestyle and dietary choices

Diagnosis and Symptoms: What Causes Kidney Disease?

Diabetes and high blood pressure are the leading causes of kidney disease in the United States, as these conditions can slowly harm the kidneys over time.

Additional causes may include autoimmune diseases that lead to gradual damage to kidney tissue, such as lupus nephritis. In some cases, the underlying cause of kidney disease remains unclear, prompting your nephrologist to recommend a kidney biopsy for further investigation.

Early Stages: A Silent Threat

Kidney disease often progresses without noticeable signs or symptoms:

- You may not feel any different until the disease reaches an advanced stage.
- Blood and urine tests are essential for determining whether you have kidney disease.
- A blood test measures your glomerular filtration rate (GFR), indicating how well your kidneys are filtering blood.
- A urine test checks for protein levels in your urine.

The Importance of Early Detection

Detecting kidney disease early can lead to effective treatment or management strategies:

- The sooner you identify kidney disease, the sooner you can initiate treatment to delay or prevent kidney failure.
- Treatments may include medications like ACE inhibitors or ARBs to manage high blood pressure, ultimately helping to preserve kidney function.

- Managing kidney disease can also reduce the risk of developing heart disease.

Long-Term Outlook

While kidney disease typically does not resolve, it can worsen over time and potentially lead to kidney failure. In such cases, treatment options include dialysis or kidney transplantation. Moreover, kidney disease can contribute to various other health conditions, including heart disease, increasing the likelihood of stroke or heart attack.

Monitoring Your Kidney Health

Many individuals with kidney disease remain asymptomatic until significant damage has occurred. Regular blood and urine tests are crucial for monitoring kidney health. These tests assess your GFR and check for albumin levels in your urine, which are fundamental in tracking the progression of kidney disease.

Key Tests to Monitor Kidney Health Include:

- Blood Pressure: Keeping your blood pressure at or below the target set by your healthcare provider is the most effective way to slow the progression of kidney disease and prevent kidney failure.

- GFR: The GFR indicates how well your kidneys filter blood. While you cannot increase your GFR, your goal should be to prevent it from declining.

- Urine Albumin: Albumin is a protein that may leak into urine when the kidneys are damaged. Although kidney damage cannot be undone, you may be able to reduce the amount of albumin in your urine through effective treatment.

- A1C: For those with diabetes, the A1C test reflects average blood glucose levels over the past three months. Lowering your A1C can significantly improve your health.

Here's a quick glance of your GFR in comparison to your Kidney Function:

STAGES OF CHRONIC KIDNEY DISEASE		GFR*	% OF KIDNEY FUNCTION
Stage 1	Kidney damage with **normal** kidney function	90 or higher	90-100%
Stage 2	Kidney damage with **mild loss** of kidney function	89 to 60	60-89%
Stage 3a	**Mild to moderate** loss of kidney function	59 to 45	45-59%
Stage 3b	**Moderate to severe** loss of kidney function	44 to 30	30-44%
Stage 4	**Severe** loss of kidney function	29 to 15	15-29%
Stage 5	Kidney **failure**	less than 15	<15%

* Your GFR number tells you how much kidney function you have left. As the kidney disease progresses, the GFR number goes down so does your kidney function.

The Role of Diet in Managing Kidney Disease

I cannot emphasize enough the critical role that renal diet foods play in managing kidney disease. Scientific consensus highlights that dietary modifications can profoundly influence the progression of Chronic Kidney Disease (CKD). Optimal nutrition—focused on a low-protein, low-sodium, and high-fiber diet—has been shown to slow the decline of kidney function. Such dietary changes not only support kidney health but also mitigate associated risks, including hypertension and diabetes. Therefore, bridging the knowledge gap in dietary management is essential for improving outcomes in CKD.

Chapter 2: The Basics of a Kidney-Friendly Diet

Key Nutrients to Monitor: Potassium, Phosphorus, Sodium, and Protein

You've probably heard it countless times, yet navigating the vast sea of dietary information can be overwhelming. If only there were a shortcut to understanding what to eat for managing chronic kidney disease (CKD)! In this chapter, I've distilled essential information into bite-sized, actionable nuggets to help you effectively manage your CKD diet.

What Should You Eat for Your CKD?

Adhering to a healthy diet is crucial for maintaining good nutritional status and slowing the progression of kidney disease. Here are key steps to follow, with a particular focus on the four essential nutrients that impact your kidney health:

1. Follow a Low-Sodium Diet and Read Labels

- Aim for a Blood Pressure Below 130/80 mmHg: Keeping your blood pressure in check is vital for kidney health.

- Limit Daily Sodium Intake: Aim for less than 2000–2300 mg of sodium per day.

- Choose Fresh and Low-Sodium Foods: Opt for fresh produce and low-sodium frozen options.

- Use Herbs for Flavor: Replace regular seasonings with herbs to enhance flavor without added sodium.

- Read Nutrition Labels: Look for sodium-free, salt-free, very low sodium, light, or reduced-sodium items instead of regular options.

2. Consume an Appropriate Amount of Protein

- Portion Control: Keep protein portions small, focusing on meat, poultry, fish, eggs, dairy, and beans.

- Consult Your Dietitian: Ask your dietitian about your specific protein needs.

- Avoid Fad Diets: Steer clear of commercial weight-loss plans like South Beach or low-carb diets.

Animal Protein Sources	Plant Protein Sources
Chicken, fish, beef, pork, lamb, eggs, dairy	Beans, nuts, lentils, tofu, grains

3. Use Healthy Cooking Methods

- Opt for Healthier Preparation: Grill, broil, bake, roast, or stir-fry instead of deep-frying.

- Trim Fat: Remove excess fat from meat and skin from poultry.

- Choose Healthy Fats: Use non-stick margarine or oils instead of butter, and select low-fat products.

Heart-Healthy Foods: Lean cuts of meat (loin or round), skinless poultry, fish, beans, vegetables, fruits, and low-fat dairy products.

4. Choose Foods with Adequate Potassium

- Monitor Potassium Intake: You may need to limit potassium as CKD progresses, especially if prescribed medications like ACE inhibitors or ARBs (Lisinopril, Avapro).

- Limit High-Potassium Foods: Avoid foods that are high in potassium.

- Skip Lite Salt: Be cautious with "lite salt" as it contains potassium instead of sodium.

- Avoid Canned Fruit/Vegetable Liquids: Don't use the liquid from canned fruits or vegetables.

- Watch Portion Sizes!

High Potassium Foods	Low Potassium Foods
Potatoes (white and sweet), tomatoes, bananas, orange juice, beans, nuts, prunes, milk, peanut butter	Apples, peaches, green beans, cauliflower, onions, celery, white bread, pasta, rice, corn flakes, rice cereal, rice milk

5. Choose Foods with Adequate Phosphorus

- Limit Phosphorus Intake: As kidney function declines, a low-phosphorus diet may be necessary to protect your bones and blood vessels.

- Watch for Phosphorus Additives: Limit dairy products, beans, lentils, nuts, organ meats, and dark colas.

- Read Ingredient Lists: Look out for "PHOS" on labels, as many packaged foods contain added phosphorus.

- Avoid Processed Meats: Choose fresh meats over deli meats that often contain phosphorus.

High Phosphorus Foods	Low Phosphorus Foods
Organ meats, dairy, beans, lentils, nuts, cola, bran cereals, oatmeal	Fresh fruits and vegetables, bread, pasta, rice milk, corn and rice cereals, light-colored soda

Hydration and Fluid Management

Chronic Kidney Disease (CKD) is classified into five stages, ranging from mild (Stage 1) to severe (Stage 5), which may require dialysis or a kidney transplant. It's crucial to note that fluid intake recommendations vary widely based on individual circumstances, including body size, activity level, climate, and other health conditions. Therefore, consider these general guidelines, but always consult your healthcare provider for personalized advice.

General Fluid Guidelines Based on CKD Stages:

- Stage 1 (GFR ≥90 mL/min): Fluid intake may not require specific restrictions unless other health conditions dictate otherwise.

Typically, healthy adults should aim for around 2 to 2.5 liters (8-10 glasses) of water per day, avoiding overconsumption.

- Stage 2 (GFR 60-89 mL/min): Similar to Stage 1, there may not be specific fluid restrictions unless necessary due to other health issues. Maintaining adequate hydration remains important.

- Stage 3 (GFR 30-59 mL/min): As kidney function declines, patients may experience fluid retention, leading to swelling and increased blood pressure. In this case, your healthcare provider may recommend limiting fluid intake.

- Stage 4 (GFR 15-29 mL/min): Significant loss of kidney filtering capacity occurs at this stage, making fluid restrictions more likely to prevent fluid overload.

- Stage 5 (GFR <15 mL/min or on dialysis): Fluid intake is usually closely monitored, especially for dialysis patients. Fluid allowances often depend on urine output and the amount of fluid removed during dialysis. It's common for hemodialysis patients to limit fluid intake to 1-1.5 liters per day.

Final Thoughts

These guidelines serve as a foundation for managing your kidney health through diet. However, individual recommendations can vary widely, so it's essential to collaborate closely with your healthcare provider to determine the appropriate dietary choices and fluid intake for your specific needs.

Chapter 3: Living Well with Kidney Disease

Myths and Facts about CKD

Despite the abundance of information available about kidney disease, many people still rely on hearsay, leading to confusion and misinformation. Here are some common myths and facts about Chronic Kidney Disease (CKD) to help clarify misunderstandings and allow you to focus on what truly matters.

Myth 1: CKD is Rare

Fact: CKD is not rare. It affects millions of people worldwide. According to the National Kidney Foundation, approximately 37 million American adults have CKD, and many are unaware of their condition.

Myth 2: There Are Clear Symptoms of CKD in the Early Stages

Fact: Most people with early-stage CKD do not exhibit clear symptoms. CKD is often referred to as a "silent" disease because it can progress without noticeable signs. This highlights the importance of regular check-ups, especially for individuals with risk factors such as diabetes, high blood pressure, or a family history of kidney disease.

Myth 3: If You Have CKD, You Will Definitely Need Dialysis or a Transplant

Fact: Not everyone with CKD progresses to kidney failure requiring dialysis or a transplant. With proper management, including lifestyle changes and medications, the progression of CKD can often be slowed or halted.

Myth 4: A High-Protein Diet is Good for Your Kidneys

Fact: A high-protein diet can actually strain your kidneys and may accelerate kidney damage in individuals with CKD. A balanced diet that includes an appropriate amount of protein is recommended.

Myth 5: Drinking More Water Will Keep Your Kidneys Healthy and Can Cure CKD

Fact: While staying hydrated is important, drinking more water than your body needs won't necessarily improve kidney function or cure CKD. In later stages of CKD, patients may need to limit fluid intake.

Myth 6: Only Adults Can Get CKD

Fact: While CKD is more common in adults, particularly older adults, children can also develop kidney disease.

Myth 7: CKD Only Happens if You Have a Pre-existing Health Condition

Fact: Although conditions like diabetes and high blood pressure significantly increase the risk of developing CKD, it can also be caused by other factors, such as certain medications, urinary tract obstructions, or inherited conditions.

Remember, if you have any questions or concerns about CKD, it's always best to consult with a healthcare provider for accurate information.

Coping Strategies

Living with Chronic Kidney Disease (CKD) presents challenges, but several strategies can help you manage the condition and maintain a good quality of life:

1. Follow Your Treatment Plan: Adhere to the treatment plan laid out by your healthcare team. This often includes managing underlying conditions like diabetes or hypertension, taking prescribed medications, following dietary guidelines, and maintaining a healthy lifestyle with regular exercise and, if applicable, smoking cessation.

2. Focus on Nutrition: Nutrition plays a vital role in managing CKD. Collaborating with a dietitian who specializes in kidney disease can be immensely beneficial. They can provide personalized advice based on your specific needs and help you navigate dietary restrictions while ensuring you receive essential nutrients.

3. Schedule Regular Check-Ups: Regular check-ups are crucial for monitoring kidney function and adjusting treatment as needed. Blood tests can help track the progression of the disease and guide necessary changes in medication or diet.

4. Manage Emotional Health: CKD can impact mental well-being, leading to feelings of anxiety, depression, or fear. Mental health professionals, such as psychologists or counselors, can provide support and teach coping strategies to manage these feelings.

5. Join a Support Group: Connecting with others who share similar experiences can provide comfort, reduce feelings of isolation, and allow for the sharing of practical advice. Organizations like the National Kidney Foundation (NKF) offer resources for finding local support groups.

6. Educate Yourself: Understanding CKD can empower you to manage your condition effectively. Reliable sources of information include your healthcare team and reputable health websites. The NKF and the American Kidney Fund offer extensive resources for patients and their families.

7. Lean on Your Support Network: Friends and family can provide emotional support, assist with practical tasks, and accompany you to medical appointments. Sharing your experiences with them can help them understand what you're going through and how they can support you.

Living with CKD requires adjustments, but with the right resources and support, patients can lead fulfilling lives while managing their condition. Always remember, you are not alone in this journey, and numerous resources are available to help.

Working with Your Healthcare Providers

Effectively collaborating with your healthcare team is crucial for managing Chronic Kidney Disease (CKD). Here are some strategies to help you maximize this relationship:

1. Open Communication: Be honest with your healthcare providers. Share all your symptoms, even those you think might not be related to your kidney disease. The more information they have, the better they can tailor your treatment plan.

2. Prepare for Appointments: Before each appointment, make a list of any questions or concerns you have. This may include new symptoms, side effects from medications, or worries about diet and lifestyle changes.

3. Understand Your Treatment Plan: Ensure you fully understand your treatment plan and the rationale behind each component. If something is unclear, don't hesitate to ask your doctor to explain it in simpler terms.

4. Role of the Dietitian: A dietitian specializing in kidney disease is an essential part of your healthcare team. They can provide personalized dietary advice based on your specific needs while helping you navigate dietary restrictions. Regularly consult with your dietitian and keep them informed about any changes in your health status.

5. Regular Monitoring: Consistent blood tests and other diagnostic evaluations are vital for tracking CKD's progression and adjusting treatment as necessary. Always attend scheduled appointments and follow through with recommended tests.

6. Follow Through: Stick to the prescribed medication regimen and dietary advice, even when you're feeling well. Consistency is key in managing CKD.

7. Share Your Feelings: Don't forget to discuss your emotional health with your healthcare team. CKD can significantly impact mental well-being, leading to anxiety or depression. There are resources available to help manage these aspects of living with a chronic illness.

8. Involve Your Family: If comfortable, consider including family members in discussions with your healthcare team. They can provide additional support, help remember information or instructions, and gain a better understanding of your experiences.

Remember, your healthcare team is there to support you in managing CKD. Reach out to them with any concerns or questions you may have; they can provide valuable guidance and resources to help you navigate this journey.

Chapter 4: Navigating High-Risk Foods & Nutrients

Now that we've covered the foods that support your health, we need to address the ones that can make your kidneys work much harder. Adjusting your diet to limit certain nutrients isn't always easy, but it's a vital part of slowing the progression of kidney disease. In this section, we'll identify the high-potassium, phosphorus, and sodium foods that typically need more oversight. Understanding why these items are restricted will help you make informed swaps and navigate your diet with much more confidence.

High-Potassium Foods

What is Potassium and Why is It Important?

Potassium is a vital mineral found in many foods, playing a crucial role in maintaining a regular heartbeat and ensuring proper muscle function. Healthy kidneys regulate potassium levels in the body, but when kidney function declines, you may need to limit foods that can elevate potassium levels to dangerous heights.

Certain medications, such as ACE inhibitors, ARBs, or diuretics like spironolactone, can also raise potassium levels. If you have high blood pressure and take these medications, keeping your potassium levels in check is critical. Symptoms of elevated potassium may include weakness, numbness, and tingling. In severe cases, dangerously high potassium can lead to irregular heartbeats or even heart attacks.

How Can You Keep Your Potassium Levels in Check?

- Limit High-Potassium Foods: Work with your renal dietitian to develop a meal plan that ensures you're getting the right amount of potassium.

- Moderation is Key: Aim for a variety of foods but in appropriate portions.

- Avoid Canned Liquid: Do not consume the liquid from canned fruits or vegetables, or juices from meats.

- Prepare Potatoes Wisely: If you want to include potatoes (which are high in potassium), peel, cut them into small pieces, soak them in water, boil, and then drain to reduce their potassium content.

- Consider Serving Sizes: Remember that nearly all foods contain some potassium; portion sizes significantly impact your overall intake. Eating a large quantity of low-potassium foods can inadvertently lead to a high-potassium meal.

What is a Safe Level of Potassium in Your Blood?

Consult your doctor or dietitian about your recent blood potassium level and record it here: _____

- SAFE Zone: 3.5 – 5.0 mg/dL

- CAUTION Zone: 5.1 – 6.0 mg/dL

- DANGER Zone: Above 6.0 mg/dL

High and Low Potassium Foods

Very High Potassium (Avoid as Much as Possible)	High Potassium (Consume Occasionally)	Low Potassium (Safe to Eat Daily)
Banana	Avocado	Apple
Orange juice	Cantaloupe, honeydew melon	Berries (strawberry, raspberries)
Prune juice	Dates, dried fruits, prunes, raisins	Cherries
Coconut milk	Kiwi, mango, orange	Grapes
Potato (white and sweet)	Artichoke, broccoli, Brussels sprouts	Peaches
Tomato and products	Dried beans, lima beans	Pear
Vegetable juice	Mushroom (canned)	Pineapple

Raisin bran cereal	Winter squash and pumpkin	Watermelon
Salt substitute (Lite salt)	Spinach and most greens (except kale)	Juices (cranberry, apple, grape)
	Organ meat	Asparagus, cucumber, eggplant
	Chocolate	Bean sprouts, green beans, green peas
		Cabbage, cauliflower, kale, lettuce
		Celery, onions, radish
		Corn, rice, noodles, pasta
		Bread and bread products
		Cereals (except raisin bran)
		Cakes, cookies (without nuts and chocolates)
		Coffee and tea

Note: High potassium foods contain more than 200 mg of potassium per serving. The serving size is typically 1/2 cup unless otherwise noted.

- Avoid very high potassium foods entirely.

- Limit high-potassium foods to two times per week, and do not consume them together on the same day.

- While meats, fish, and poultry are high in potassium, they are essential for maintaining good nutritional status, so include them in your diet as needed.

Low potassium foods contain less than 200 mg of potassium per serving (1/2 cup unless otherwise noted). You can enjoy these foods daily, but always be mindful of portion sizes.

High-Phosphorus Foods

What is Phosphorus?

Phosphorus is a mineral crucial for building strong bones and maintaining overall health, working alongside calcium.

Why is Phosphorus Important?

Healthy kidneys can effectively remove excess phosphorus from your blood. However, when you have chronic kidney disease, your kidneys struggle to eliminate phosphorus, leading to elevated levels that can cause significant health issues. High phosphorus can pull calcium from your bones, weakening them and causing dangerous deposits in your blood vessels, lungs, eyes, and heart. Therefore, managing phosphorus levels is vital for your overall health.

What is a Safe Blood Level of Phosphorus?

A normal phosphorus level ranges from 2.1 to 4.6 mg/dL. Consult your doctor or dietitian regarding your last phosphorus level and record it here: _____.

How Can I Control My Phosphorus Level?

You can maintain normal phosphorus levels through dietary management and medications. Work closely with your dietitian and doctor to create a plan. Below is a list of foods high in phosphorus that you should limit or avoid:

High Phosphorus Foods to Limit or Avoid:

Food Category	Foods to Avoid
Beverages	Ale, beer, chocolate drinks, cocoa, milk-based drinks, canned iced tea, dark colas
Dairy Products	Cheese, custard, milk, cream soups, cottage cheese, ice cream, pudding, yogurt
Protein	Beef liver, fish roe, oysters, crayfish, chicken liver, organ meats, sardines

Vegetables	Dried beans and peas (baked beans, black beans, chickpeas, kidney beans, lima beans, lentils, northern beans, split peas, soybeans)
Others	Bran cereals, brewer's yeast, caramels, nuts, seeds, wheat germ, whole grain products

What Should I Do If My Phosphorus Level is Too High?

If your phosphorus level is elevated, consider selecting foods from the low-phosphorus list. Discuss dietary changes with your dietitian and doctor, and inquire about phosphate binder prescriptions.

High Phosphorus Foods and Alternatives:

Instead of	Phos (mg)	Low Phosphorus Foods	Phos (mg)
8 oz milk	230	8 oz non-dairy creamer or 4 oz milk	110 115
8 oz cream soup (with milk)	275	8 oz cream soup (with water)	90
1 oz hard cheese	145	1 oz cream cheese	30
1/2 cup ice cream	80	1/2 cup sorbet or 1 popsicle	0
1/2 cup lima or pinto beans	100	1/2 cup mixed vegetables (green beans)	35
12 oz can cola	55	12 oz ginger ale or lemon soda	3
1/2 cup custard (with milk)	150	1/2 cup pudding (made with non-dairy creamer)	50
2 oz peanuts	200	1 1/2 cup light or low-fat popcorn	35
1 1/2 oz chocolate bar	125	1 1/2 oz hard candy (fruit flavors or jelly beans)	3

2/3 cup oatmeal	130	2/3 cup cream of wheat or grits	40
1/2 cup bran cereal	140-260	1/2 cup non-bran cereal (shredded wheat, rice cereals, or cornflakes)	50-100

High-Sodium Foods

What is Sodium?

Sodium is a mineral that naturally occurs in foods and is the primary component of table salt.

Why Should I Limit My Sodium Intake?

While some sodium is necessary for maintaining water balance in the body, excessive sodium intake can exacerbate conditions like high blood pressure and congestive heart failure, leading to:

- Increased thirst

- Fluid retention

- Elevated blood pressure

Reducing sodium in your diet can help manage these issues.

Tips to Cut Down Sodium Intake

- Cook with Herbs and Spices: Replace salt with herbs and spices for flavor.

- Read Food Labels: Choose foods low in sodium.

- Avoid Salt Substitutes: Steer clear of low-sodium products made with salt substitutes, as they often contain high potassium levels.

- Dining Out: Request meats or fish without added salt, and ask for sauces or gravies on the side, as they may contain large amounts of salt.

Food	Avoid	Choose
Dairy	Buttermilk, Cottage cheese, regular cheese	2%, 1% or skim milk, low fat yogurt, low sodium cheese
Meats	**Processed and luncheon meats** Ham, bacon, salt pork, sausage Hotdogs, corned beef, Spam , Pastrami **Breaded or fried meats** Chicken, fish pork or beef **Canned meats in oil** Sardines, salmon, tuna	Fresh beef, veal, pork, poultry, fish, eggs Low-salt deli meat
Starches	Salted crackers or bread, Pretzels Potato chips, corn chips, tortilla chips, popcorn Instant mashed potatoes Mixed muffins, pancakes, potatoes, noodles, some dry cereals	Fresh bread, most commercial bread Unsalted chips, crackers, pretzels Read labels for dry cereals Unsalted popcorn
Vegetables	Canned vegetables Pickles, sauerkraut, olives, relish, vegetable juice, vegetable soup tomato products Frozen vegetables with cheese or cream sauces	All plain fresh and frozen vegetables Low-sodium canned vegetables Low-sodium tomato sauces Homemade or low-sodium soups
Fruits	None	All
Condiments	Table salt, garlic salt, celery salt Lite salt, Bouillon cubes, seasoning salt, onion salt, lemon pepper, meat tenderizer, flavored enhancers, salt	Fresh garlic, fresh onion, garlic powder, onion powder, black

	substitutes, catsup/ketchup, mustard, salad dressing, soy sauce, steak sauce, barbecue sauce, teriyaki sauce, oyster sauce, hot sauce, Worcestershire sauce	pepper, lemon juice, low-sodium or salt-free seasoning blends, vinegar, homemade or low sodium sauces and salad dressings, dry mustard
Others	**Convenience foods** TV dinners, Chili, spaghetti, frozen prepared foods, fast foods, canned raviolis, macaroni & cheese **Most Chinese, Mexican, and Pizza restaurants**	Low sodium frozen dinner, home-made casseroles without added salt, soups made with fresh or raw vegetables, fresh meat, rice, pasta or unsalted canned vegetables Request no salt on foods when eating out. Ask for sauces on the side when dinning out.

Understanding Nutrition Labels

To help you keep sodium in check, understanding nutrition labels is essential. This knowledge will also assist you in monitoring potassium and protein content.

	New Label	Current Label
Check Serving Size	**Nutrition Facts** 8 servings per container **Serving size 2/3 cup (55g)**	**Nutrition Facts** Serving Size 2/3 cup (55g) Servings Per Container About 8
Check Calories	**Amount per serving** **Calories 230**	**Amount Per Serving** **Calories** 230 Calories from Fat 72
Limit These Nutrients	% Daily Value* Total Fat 8g 10% Saturated Fat 1g 5% Trans Fat 0g Cholesterol 0mg 0% Sodium 160mg 7% Total Carbohydrate 37g 13% Dietary Fiber 4g 14%	% Daily Value* **Total Fat** 8g 12% Saturated Fat 1g 5% Trans Fat 0g **Cholesterol** 0mg 0% **Sodium** 160mg 7% **Total Carbohydrate** 37g 12% Dietary Fiber 4g 16% Sugars 1g **Protein** 3g
Get Enough of These Nutrients	Total Sugars 12g Includes 10g Added Sugars 20% Protein 3g	Vitamin A 10% Vitamin C 8% Calcium 20% Iron 45%
Watch for Potassium	Vitamin D 2mcg 10% Calcium 260mg 20% Iron 8mg 45% Potassium 235mg 6% * The % Daily Value (DV) tells you how much a nutrient in a serving of food contributes to a daily diet. 2,000 calories a day is used for general nutrition advice.	* Percent Daily Values are based on a 2,000 calorie diet. Your daily value may be higher or lower depending on your calorie needs.

1. Portion Check: Look at the serving size and the number of servings per container. For example, if one serving is ⅔ cup, eating the entire package amounts to about 5 cups.

2. Calorie Control: Calories reflect the energy you receive per serving. For instance, if one serving provides 230 calories, consuming the entire package results in 1840 calories.

    •   General Guidelines: Low = 50 calories per serving; High = 400 calories per serving.

3. Limit These Nutrients:

    •   Saturated fat, trans fat, sodium, and added sugars.

    •   Low Fat: 3 g or less of total fat per serving.

    •   Low Sodium: 140 mg or less per serving; it's acceptable to choose items with less than 200 mg.

4. Get Enough of These Nutrients:

- Look for foods rich in fiber, protein, and essential vitamins and minerals.

- Key nutrients include:

    - Vitamin D, Calcium, and Iron

    - Fiber: 3 g or more per serving is good; 5 g or more is high.

    - Protein: Vital for energy, muscle maintenance, and wound healing. Consult your doctor or dietitian regarding your specific protein needs.

5. Watch for Potassium:

- Based on your individual requirements, aim for low-potassium choices (less than 200 mg per serving). Discuss your potassium needs with your dietitian.

Chapter 5: Meal Planning for Kidney Health

Creating a Balanced Meal Plan

Developing a balanced meal plan for individuals with Chronic Kidney Disease (CKD) can be challenging due to the varying dietary requirements at each stage of the disease. However, it's essential to remember that every patient is unique, and these guidelines should be customized to meet individual needs and circumstances. Always consult with a healthcare provider or a renal dietitian before making any changes to your diet. In the following chapters, I will provide carefully selected CKD recipes, but for now, here are general daily meal plan guidelines for each CKD stage:

Stage 1 and 2 Chronic Kidney Disease (CKD) Daily Meal Plan Guidelines

Patients with Stage 1 and 2 CKD typically do not need to follow a strict renal diet. Instead, they should focus on a healthy, balanced diet that promotes overall health and slows disease progression.

The dietary guidelines below are general in nature, as individual needs can vary greatly based on age, sex, weight, physical activity level, and other health conditions. It's crucial to consult with a healthcare provider or a registered dietitian for personalized advice.

Caloric Intake

Maintaining a balanced caloric intake is vital for sustaining a healthy weight. The daily caloric requirement varies based on individual factors, but here is a general guideline:

- For Men: 2000 - 2500 calories per day

- For Women: 1600 - 2000 calories per day

Proteins

Protein is essential for growth, repair, and overall health. However, excessive protein intake can put additional strain on the kidneys. The recommended daily protein intake for CKD Stage 1 and 2 is approximately:

- 0.8 grams of protein per kilogram of body weight.

Carbohydrates

Carbohydrates serve as the body's primary energy source. Choose complex carbohydrates such as whole grains, fruits, and vegetables over simple sugars.

- Aim for about 45-65% of your daily caloric intake from carbohydrates.

Fats

Healthy fats are vital for heart health. Opt for unsaturated fats found in fish, nuts, seeds, avocados, and olives.

- Aim for about 20-35% of your daily caloric intake from fats.

Sample Meal Plan for Stages 1 and 2

Here's a sample meal plan that aligns with these guidelines:

Breakfast:

- ☼ 1 cup cooked oatmeal topped with a sprinkle of nuts
- ☼ 1 medium-sized banana
- ☼ 1 cup of skim milk or a dairy alternative

Lunch:

- ☼ 2 oz grilled chicken breast
- ☼ 1 cup steamed vegetables (such as broccoli or cauliflower)
- ☼ 1/2 cup cooked brown rice

Afternoon Snack:

- ☼ 1 small apple
- ☼ A handful of unsalted almonds

Dinner:

- ☼ 3 oz baked salmon
- ☼ 1 cup roasted sweet potato
- ☼ Side salad with mixed greens, tomatoes, cucumber, and a drizzle of olive oil dressing

Evening Snack:

- ☼ 1 cup low-fat yogurt topped with a sprinkle of berries

Remember to stay hydrated and limit your sodium intake, as excessive sodium can raise blood pressure and cause fluid retention, both of which can exacerbate kidney disease.

As CKD progresses to later stages (3 to 5), dietary needs will change significantly, often requiring decreased intake of protein, potassium, phosphorus, and sodium. Regular monitoring and consultation with healthcare providers are crucial.

Stage 3-5 Chronic Kidney Disease (CKD) Daily Meal Plan Guidelines

As kidney function declines in the later stages of CKD (Stages 3 to 5), the kidneys struggle to remove waste products from protein metabolism, necessitating a reduction in protein intake. Additionally, potassium, phosphorus, and sodium levels must be carefully monitored and limited.

These meal plans are general guidelines. Individual needs can vary greatly, so always consult with a healthcare provider or a registered dietitian for personalized advice.

Stage 3 CKD Daily Nutrient Requirements

- Caloric Intake:

    - For Men: 2000 - 2500 calories per day

    - For Women: 1600 - 2000 calories per day

- Proteins:

    - Approximately 0.8 grams per kilogram of body weight.

- Carbohydrates:

    - Aim for about 45-65% of your daily caloric intake from carbohydrates.

- Fats:

    - Aim for about 20-35% of your daily caloric intake from fats.

- Sodium:

    - Aim for less than 2000 mg per day.

- Potassium and Phosphorus:

    - Your healthcare provider will advise you based on your blood levels.

Stage 3 CKD Sample Meal Plan

Breakfast:

- ✿ 1 cup of cream of wheat
- ✿ 1 slice of toast with 1 tablespoon of jelly
- ✿ 1 small apple
- ✿ 1 cup of coffee or tea

Lunch:

- ✿ Turkey sandwich: 2 oz turkey on whole grain bread with lettuce and mayonnaise
- ✿ 15 grapes
- ✿ Water or unsweetened iced tea

Afternoon Snack:

- ✿ 1 medium-sized peach
- ✿ A handful of rice cakes

Dinner:

- ✿ 3 oz grilled chicken breast
- ✿ 1 cup of cooked zucchini
- ✿ 1/2 cup of white rice
- ✿ Water or homemade lemonade (watching for sugar content)

Evening Snack:

- ✿ 1 cup of low-fat vanilla yogurt

Stage 4 CKD Daily Nutrient Requirements

- Caloric Intake:
    - For Men: 2000 - 2500 calories per day
    - For Women: 1600 - 2000 calories per day
- Proteins:
    - Approximately 0.6 grams per kilogram of body weight.
- Carbohydrates:
    - Aim for about 45-65% of your daily caloric intake from carbohydrates.
- Fats:
    - Aim for about 20-35% of your daily caloric intake from fats.
- Sodium:
    - Aim for less than 2000 mg per day.
- Potassium and Phosphorus:
    - Your healthcare provider will advise you based on your blood levels, often recommending potassium to be limited to 2000-3000 mg per day and phosphorus to less than 800-1000 mg per day.

Stage 4 CKD Sample Meal Plan

Breakfast:

- 1/2 cup high-protein cereal with almond milk
- 1 slice of toast with margarine
- 1/2 cup fresh blueberries
- Coffee or tea

Lunch:

- Tuna salad (made with low-sodium canned tuna) on a bed of lettuce
- Sliced cucumber and cherry tomatoes

- ✿ 1/2 cup applesauce
- ✿ Water or unsweetened iced tea

Afternoon Snack:

- ✿ Rice cakes with a thin layer of cream cheese
- ✿ 1/2 cup fresh pineapple chunks

Dinner:

- ✿ 3 oz baked fish (like cod)
- ✿ 1 cup steamed green beans
- ✿ 1/2 cup mashed cauliflower
- ✿ Water or cranberry juice (unsweetened)

Evening Snack:

- ✿ 2 cups air-popped popcorn

Stage 5 CKD Daily Nutrient Requirements (Not on Dialysis)

- Caloric Intake:
    - For Men: 2000 - 2500 calories per day
    - For Women: 1600 - 2000 calories per day
- Proteins:
    - Approximately 0.6 grams per kilogram of body weight.
- Carbohydrates:
    - Aim for about 45-65% of your daily caloric intake from carbohydrates.
- Fats:
    - Aim for about 20-35% of your daily caloric intake from fats.
- Sodium:
    - Aim for less than 2000 mg per day.
- Potassium and Phosphorus:
    - Your healthcare provider will advise you based on your blood levels, often recommending potassium to be limited to 2000-3000 mg per day and phosphorus to less than 800-1000 mg per day.

Stage 5 CKD Sample Meal Plan

Breakfast:

- 1/2 cup cream of wheat
- White toast with jelly
- 1/2 cup sliced peaches (canned in juice, not syrup)
- Coffee or tea

Lunch:

- Egg salad sandwich: 1 boiled egg on white bread with lettuce and mayonnaise

- ☼ Apple slices
- ☼ Water or homemade lemonade (watching for sugar content)

Afternoon Snack:

- ☼ Rice cakes
- ☼ 15 fresh grapes

Dinner:

- ☼ 2 oz roasted chicken
- ☼ 1/2 cup cooked carrots
- ☼ 1/2 cup white rice
- ☼ Water or cranberry juice (unsweetened)

Evening Snack:

- ☼ 5 vanilla wafers

These meal plans aim to restrict protein, potassium, phosphorus, and sodium intake while providing adequate calories and other nutrients. However, dietary restrictions may vary based on specific lab results. Remember, these are general guidelines, and individual needs can differ significantly based on factors like age, sex, weight, physical activity level, and overall health. Always consult with a healthcare provider for personalized advice.

Portion Control and Serving Sizes

What Distinguishes a Portion from a Serving?

A portion refers to the quantity of food you choose to consume in one sitting, whether at a restaurant, from a packaged product, or at your own dining table. In contrast, a serving size is the specific amount of food defined on a product's Nutrition Facts label.

Serving sizes can vary across different products and may be measured in various units such as cups, ounces, grams, or countable units (like three crackers). Your chosen portion size may align with or differ from the listed serving size based on your appetite.

To determine how many servings are in a container, check the top of the label where "Servings per container" is stated just above "Serving size." For instance, if a frozen lasagna lists 1 cup as the serving size and contains four servings per container, consuming 2 cups (or half the package) means you're eating two servings, which would double the calories and other nutrients listed on the food label.

- Example Calculation:
    - 1 serving = 280 calories
    - 2 servings = 280 × 2 = 560 calories

It's crucial to consult with your doctor and dietitian to determine your daily requirements for protein, sodium, potassium, and phosphorus. Your needs may vary based on:

- Age
- Current weight and height
- Metabolism
- Gender
- Activity level
- Lab numbers

As a CKD patient, always compare general guidelines with what your healthcare team prescribes. To aid in this process, I've created a "Handy" food portioning guide in collaboration with Covenant Home Care to assist my patients.

"Handy" Guide to Correct Food Portions

We often know what to eat but not how much. It turns out that whether you are a man or woman, big or small, your own hand is the perfect measuring device for you. Follow this handy guide to determine correct food portions for your next meal. *Source: Arizona State University School of Nutrition & Health Promotion*

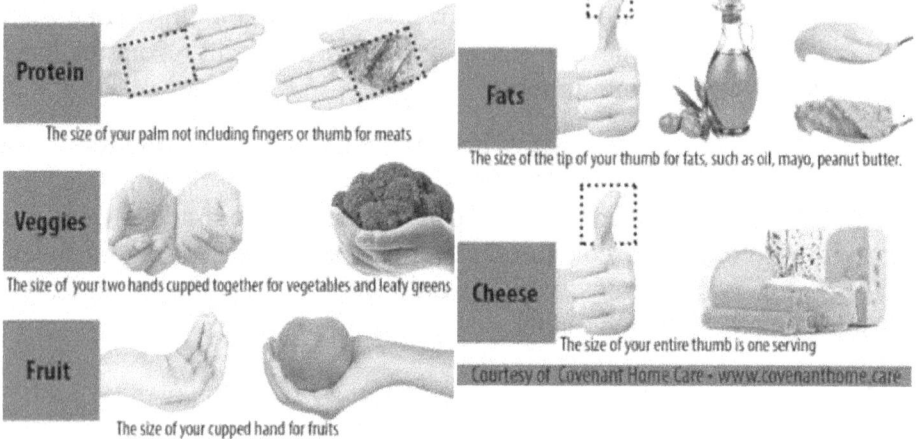

Starches
The size of your fist for starches, such as rice, potatoes, pasta

Protein
The size of your palm not including fingers or thumb for meats

Fats
The size of the tip of your thumb for fats, such as oil, mayo, peanut butter.

Veggies
The size of your two hands cupped together for vegetables and leafy greens

Cheese
The size of your entire thumb is one serving

Courtesy of Covenant Home Care • www.covenanthome.care

Fruit
The size of your cupped hand for fruits

Tips For Grocery Shopping

The grocery store is your gateway to a diverse selection of food that can contribute to your well-being, especially when living with chronic kidney disease (CKD). Making informed choices here can significantly influence your health. Here are eight tips to help you navigate your grocery shopping experience:

1. Check the Quality Before Buying: Fresh and nutritious foods tend to last longer than their less healthy counterparts. Examine fruits and vegetables for quality before purchasing. If they appear wilted or unusually discolored, opt for fresher options. Seasonal produce often provides the best flavor and affordability.

2. Avoid Processed Foods: Grocery stores offer a mix of healthful and less healthful options. To avoid processed foods, bypass candy and sugary snacks in favor of fresh fruits and vegetables. Look for minimally processed alternatives, typically found in the natural food sections.

3. Don't Shop on an Empty Stomach: Hunger can influence your shopping habits, leading you to purchase items you wouldn't normally choose due to diminished willpower. Try to avoid shopping when you're feeling hungry.

4. Write Down a Grocery List and Stick with It: Creating a detailed grocery list before you shop can help ensure that you only buy what you need, preventing impulse purchases of unhealthy items. Use paper or a digital note-taking app for convenience. With a meal plan in place, your shopping list is already prepared!

5. Buy Whole Foods: Whole foods—those in their most natural state without added artificial flavors, sweeteners, or preservatives—are the best choice. Studies indicate that individuals who consume more whole foods have a lower body mass index (BMI) and are less likely to develop heart disease and diabetes. Avoid processed and packaged foods that contain unnecessary additives and fillers, which can add calories without contributing nutritional value.

Chapter 6. Renal Diet Recipes

Breakfast Dishes

Kidney Friendly Smoothies

GREEN DETOX SMOOTHIE			
Servings:	2	Preparation Time	10 minutes

INGREDIENTS	DIRECTIONS
1 cup Romaine lettuce 1 cucumber (chopped) 1/2 lemon (juiced) 1 pears (peeled and chopped) 1 tbsp ginger (grated) 1 tbsp ground flax seed 1 1/2 cups water 5 Ice cubes	1. Place all ingredients together in a blender. Blend until smooth. Be patient! No one likes clumps in their smoothies. It may take 1 minute or longer to get a great, smoothie-consistency. 2. Divide between glasses and enjoy!

NUTRIENT FACTS	TOTAL	PER SERVING
Calories (kCal):	164	82
Proteins (g):	4	2
Carbohydrates (g):	38	19
Fats (g):	2	1
Potassium (mg):	647	323.5
Phosphorus (mg):	100	50
Sodium (mg):	11.24	5.62

FRESH MANGO SMOOTHIE

Servings:	2	Preparation Time	10 minutes

INGREDIENTS	DIRECTIONS
1/2 cup frozen mango 1/2 cup frozen cauliflower 1 banana (medium) 1 1/2 cup water 1 1/2 tsp apple cider vinegar	1. Place all ingredients in your blender and blend until smooth. Pour into a glass and enjoy!

NUTRIENT FACTS	TOTAL	PER SERVING
Calories (kCal):	173	86.5
Proteins (g):	3	1.5
Carbohydrates (g):	43	21.5
Fats (g):	1	0.5
Potassium (mg):	648	324
Phosphorus (mg):	57	28.5
Sodium (mg):	17	8.5

BREAKFAST TRAIL MIX

Servings:	3	Preparation Time	5 mins or less

INGREDIENTS	DIRECTIONS
1 cup Corn cereal 1 cup Rice cereal 1/2 cup Cocoa cereal 1/2 cup mini rice cakes (plain or apple cinnamon)	1. Mix all ingredients together in a medium bowl then divide into 1 cup portions. 2. Serve dry or with your preferred milk.

NUTRIENT FACTS	TOTAL	PER SERVING
Calories (kCal):	145	48.33
Proteins (g):	2	0.67
Carbohydrates (g):	32	10.67
Fats (g):	1	0.33
Potassium (mg):	210	70
Phosphorus (mg):	150	50
Sodium (mg):	600	200

GRANOLA IN YOGURT & APPLESAUCE

Servings:	1	Preparation Time	5 mins

INGREDIENTS	DIRECTIONS
1/2 cup plain greek yogurt 1/4 cup unsweetened applesauce 1/4 cup granola 2 tbsps. pumpkin seeds	1. Mix the yogurt and apple sauce together in a bowl. 2. Top with granola and pumpkin seeds. Enjoy!

NUTRIENT FACTS	TOTAL	PER SERVING
Calories (kCal):	355	355
Proteins (g):	20	20
Carbohydrates (g):	31	31
Fats (g):	18	18
Potassium (mg):	336	336
Phosphorus (mg):	347	347
Sodium (mg):	196	196

GUACAMOLE DIP & PLANTAIN CHIPS

Servings:	4	Preparation Time	10 mins

INGREDIENTS	DIRECTIONS
1 avocado (medium, ripe) 2 tbsps. nutritional yeast 1 tbsp lemon juice 1/4 tsp sea salt 1/2 cup plantain chips (store-bought or homemade)	1. In a bowl, mash together the avocado, nutritional yeast, lemon juice, and sea salt with a fork. 2. Place the guacamole in a bowl and serve with plantain chips. Enjoy!

NUTRIENT FACTS	TOTAL	PER SERVING
Calories (kCal):	247	61.75
Proteins (g):	7	1.75
Carbohydrates (g):	18	4.5
Fats (g):	18	4.5
Potassium (mg):	1470	367.5
Phosphorus (mg):	98	24.5
Sodium (mg):	611	152.75

Note:

1/2 cup plantain chips (store-bought or homemade): The content can vary greatly depending on the brand used. On average it might contain approximately 400mg of potassium, negligible amounts of phosphorus, and ~10-20mg of sodium.

Lunch Dishes

Light and Nourishing Salads

FARRO AND CHICKPEA BOWL

Servings:	3	Preparation Time	25 mins

INGREDIENTS	DIRECTIONS
1 1/2 cup chickpeas (cooked) 2 tbsps. balsamic vinegar 1 tbsp maple syrup (to taste) 1/2 cup chives (chopped) pinch of sea salt & black pepper (to taste) 1/2 cup farro (rinsed) 1/4 cup pesto 1 cup cherry tomatoes 1 tbsp avocado oil	1. Combine the chickpeas, balsamic vinegar, maple syrup, chives, salt, and pepper in a bowl. Set aside. 2. Meanwhile, cook the farro according to the package directions. 3. Stir in the pesto. Set aside. 4. Toss the tomatoes in oil, salt, and pepper on a baking sheet. 5. Broil for six to eight minutes on the middle rack. 6. Divide the farro, chickpeas, and tomatoes evenly between bowls. Enjoy!

NUTRIENT FACTS	TOTAL	PER SERVING
Calories (kCal):	415	138.33
Proteins (g):	15	5
Carbohydrates (g):	54	18
Fats (g):	16	5.33
Potassium (mg):	1090	363.33
Phosphorus (mg):	382	127.33
Sodium (mg):	512	170.67

PASTA SALAD NIÇOISE

Servings:	6	Preparation Time Chill Time	25 mins 1-2 hrs

INGREDIENTS

4 cups cooked small shell macaroni
1 tablespoon olive oil
2 cups fresh green beans, cut in 1-inch pieces
1 /2 cup lemon juice
1 /3 cup olive oil
2 teaspoons dry mustard
1 tablespoon chopped fresh parsley
1 teaspoon basil
1 7-3/4-oz can tuna packed in water, drained
5 green onions, chopped, including tops
1 /4 teaspoon pepper

DIRECTIONS

1. Combine the chickpeas, balsamic vinegar, maple syrup, chives, salt, and pepper in a bowl. Set aside.
2. Meanwhile, cook the farro according to the package directions.
3. Stir in the pesto. Set aside.
4. Toss the tomatoes in oil, salt, and pepper on a baking sheet.
5. Broil for six to eight minutes on the middle rack.
6. Divide the farro, chickpeas, and tomatoes evenly between bowls. Enjoy!

NUTRIENT FACTS

	TOTAL	PER SERVING
Calories (kCal):	304	50.67
Proteins (g):	15	2.50
Carbohydrates (g):	25	4.17
Fats (g):	16	2.67
Potassium (mg):	1545	257.50
Phosphorus (mg):	519	86.50
Sodium (mg):	381	63.50

BLUEBERRY COCONUT CREPES

Servings:	3	Preparation Time	15 mins

INGREDIENTS

1/4 cup canned coconut milk
1/4 cup frozen blueberries
4 eggs (large)
3 tbsps. coconut flour
1/8 tsp sea salt
2 tbsps. coconut oil (divided)

DIRECTIONS

1. Add the coconut milk, blueberries, eggs, coconut flour, and salt to a blender. Blend until smooth.
2. Heat a bit of the coconut oil in a skillet over medium heat.
3. Pour 1/4 cup of the batter at a time and gently swirl to spread it into a thin layer. Cook each side for about 30 seconds to one minute.
4. Repeat with the remaining batter and coconut oil.
5. Divide the crepes onto plates and enjoy!

NUTRIENT FACTS	TOTAL	PER SERVING
Calories (kCal):	248.01	82.67
Proteins (g):	9.99	3.33
Carbohydrates (g):	6.99	2.33
Fats (g):	20.01	6.67
Potassium (mg):	373.98	124.66
Phosphorus (mg):	567.99	189.33
Sodium (mg):	604.02	201.34

STACKED VEGETABLE SANDWICH

Servings:	1	Preparation Time	5 mins

INGREDIENTS

2 tbsps. hummus
2 slices whole grain bread
1/16 green lettuce (leaves separated)
1/4 tomato (medium, sliced)
1/4 cup radishes (trimmed, sliced)
1 tbsp red onion (sliced)
1/2 carrot (small, shredded)

DIRECTIONS

1. Spread the hummus on the bread.
2. Add the remaining sandwich toppings.
3. Close the sandwich and enjoy!

NUTRIENT FACTS	TOTAL	PER SERVING
Calories (kCal):	317	317
Proteins (g):	14	14
Carbohydrates (g):	46	46
Fats (g):	9	9
Potassium (mg):	567	567
Phosphorus (mg):	177	177
Sodium (mg):	476	476

Dinner Dishes

Main Course

LEMON, GARLIC, & HERB PASTA

Servings:	3	Preparation Time	20 mins

INGREDIENTS	DIRECTIONS
2 cups brown rice penne (uncooked) 2 cups chickpeas (cooked, drained) 1 tbsp extra virgin olive oil 1 1/2 tbsp lemon juice 2 garlic cloves (minced) 1/2 tsp oregano pinch of sea salt & black pepper (to taste) 2 tbsps. parsley (chopped) 2 tbsps. basil leaves (chopped) 2 tbsps. fresh dill (chopped) Note: Pinch = 1/16 teaspoon	1. Cook pasta according to the package. 2. While the pasta is cooking, in a bowl, add the chickpeas, olive oil, lemon juice, garlic, oregano, salt and pepper. Mix to combine and set aside to marinate. 3. Add the pasta to a serving bowl followed by the chickpea mix (including the liquid). 4. Toss to combine. Add the parsley, basil, dill and toss again. Divide into bowls and enjoy!

NUTRIENT FACTS	TOTAL	PER SERVING
Calories (kCal):	506	168.67
Proteins (g):	15	5
Carbohydrates (g):	89	29.67
Fats (g):	10	3.33
Potassium (mg):	1087	362.33
Phosphorus (mg):	622	207.33
Sodium (mg):	182	60.67

COUSCOUS & MUSHROOM BOWL

Servings: 2	Preparation Time	25 mins

INGREDIENTS

2 eggs
2 tsps. extra virgin olive oil (divided)
1 cup Israeli couscous
2 cups water
2 tbsps. shallots (peeled, chopped)
2 garlic cloves (minced)
6 cremini mushrooms (sliced)
Pinch of sea salt & black pepper (to taste)

Note: Pinch = 1/16 teaspoon

DIRECTIONS

1. Place eggs in a saucepan and cover with water. Bring to a boil over high heat. Once
boiling, turn off the heat but keep the saucepan on the hot burner. Cover and let sit
for 10 to 12 minutes.
2. Strain the water and fill the saucepan with cold water. Once cooled, peel, halve and set aside.
3. Heat half the oil in a saucepan over medium heat. Add the couscous and toast for one
to two minutes, stirring often.
4. Pour in the water and bring to a simmer and cook for 8 to 10 minutes, until cooked through. Drain excess water and set aside.
5. In a skillet over medium-low heat, pour in the remaining oil. Add the shallot and sauté
until softened, about three minutes.
6. Then add the garlic and mushrooms and continue cooking until the mushrooms are cooked through and water is released, about five minutes.
7. Divide the couscous into bowls and top with mushrooms and the egg. Season with salt
and pepper. Enjoy!

NUTRIENT FACTS	TOTAL	PER SERVING
Calories (kCal):	393	196.5
Proteins (g):	17	8.5
Carbohydrates (g):	59	29.5
Fats (g):	9	4.5
Potassium (mg):	530	265
Phosphorus (mg):	342	171
Sodium (mg):	304	152

Side Dish

HALLOUMI MUSHROOM TACOS

Servings:	2	Preparation Time	20 mins

INGREDIENTS

1 tsp extra virgin olive oil
6 cremini mushrooms (sliced)
pinch of sea salt & black pepper
(to taste)
2.5 ozs halloumi (sliced)
1/2 cup pineapple (chopped)
2 tbsps. cilantro (chopped)
2 tbsps. lime juice
4 corn tortillas

Note: Pinch = 1/16 teaspoon

DIRECTIONS

1. Heat the oil in a pan over medium-high heat. Add the mushrooms and cook for three to five minutes or until golden brown. Season with salt and pepper. Remove and set them aside.
2. In a small bowl, mix together the pineapple, cilantro, and lime juice.
3. Divide the mushrooms and halloumi between the tortillas.
4. Top with pineapple salsa, season with additional salt and pepper if needed, and enjoy!
5. In the same pan, cook the halloumi slices until golden brown, about one to two minutes per side.

NUTRIENT FACTS	TOTAL	PER SERVING
Calories (kCal):	475	237.50
Proteins (g):	22	11
Carbohydrates (g):	36	18
Fats (g):	26	13
Potassium (mg):	604	302
Phosphorus (mg):	809	404.50
Sodium (mg):	905	452.5

FRESH FRUIT AND SWEET CRANBERRY DIP

Servings:	24	Preparation Time	10 mins
		Chill time	At least 30 mins

INGREDIENTS

8 ounces sour cream
1/2 cup whole berry cranberry sauce
1/4 teaspoon nutmeg
1/4 teaspoon ground ginger
4 medium pears, sliced into 12 slices each
4 medium apples, cut into 12 slices each
4 cups fresh pineapple, cut into bite-size pieces
1 teaspoon lemon juice

DIRECTIONS

1. Put sour cream, cranberry sauce, nutmeg and ground ginger in a food processor. It should be well-mixed, then transfer to a small bowl.
2. Then, cut the fresh fruit into small pieces. To prevent browning, toss apple and pear with lemon juice.
3. For final touches, arrange the fruits on platter with dip bowl then chill until ready.

NUTRIENT FACTS	TOTAL	PER SERVING
Calories (kCal):	70	2.92
Proteins (g):	0	0
Carbohydrates (g):	13	0.54
Fats (g):	2	0.08
Potassium (mg):	2791	116.29
Phosphorus (mg):	320	13.33
Sodium (mg):	129	5.38

Snacks

LEMON, GARLIC, & HERB PASTA

Servings:	3	Preparation Time	20 mins

INGREDIENTS	DIRECTIONS
2 cups brown rice penne (uncooked) 2 cups chickpeas (cooked, drained) 1 tbsp extra virgin olive oil 1 1/2 tbsp lemon juice 2 garlic cloves (minced) 1/2 tsp oregano pinch of sea salt & black pepper (to taste) 2 tbsps. parsley (chopped) 2 tbsps. basil leaves (chopped) 2 tbsps. fresh dill (chopped) Note: Pinch = 1/16 teaspoon	1. Cook pasta according to the package. 2. While the pasta is cooking, in a bowl, add the chickpeas, olive oil, lemon juice, garlic, oregano, salt and pepper. Mix to combine and set aside to marinate. 3. Add the pasta to a serving bowl followed by the chickpea mix (including the liquid). 4. Toss to combine. Add the parsley, basil, dill and toss again. Divide into bowls and enjoy!

NUTRIENT FACTS	TOTAL	PER SERVING
Calories (kCal):	506	**168.67**
Proteins (g):	15	**5**
Carbohydrates (g):	89	**29.67**
Fats (g):	10	**3.33**
Potassium (mg):	1087	**362.33**
Phosphorus (mg):	622	**207.33**
Sodium (mg):	182	**60.67**

CHOCOLATE PEANUT BUTTER MUFFIN

Servings:	9	Preparation Time	40 mins

INGREDIENTS

3 bananas (medium, ripe, mashed)

3 eggs

1/3 cup maple syrup

1/2 tsp vanilla extract

3 tbsps. Coconut oil

1/2 tsp sea salt

1 cup all natural peanut butter (divided)

1/2 tsp baking soda

1 tsp baking powder

1/2 cup cacao powder

DIRECTIONS

1. Preheat the oven to 375°F (190°C). Line a muffin tray with liners or use a silicone muffin tray.
2. Mix the mashed banana and egg together. Using a hand mixer or stand mixer is best, but a whisk will also work.
3. Slowly add the maple syrup and vanilla and continue mixing. Next, add the oil until an even consistency is achieved.
4. Add the salt and 3/4 of the peanut butter. Continue to mix, then add the baking soda and baking powder. Slowly add the cacao powder. Continue to mix until a pancake batter-like consistency is achieved.
5. Fill each muffin liner with the batter, approximately 1/3 cup each. Add the remaining peanut butter onto the top of each muffin and if desired, swirl with a toothpick.
6. Bake in the oven for 25 minutes or until muffin tops are firm. Remove from the oven, allow to cool in the muffin tin for 10 minutes before removing. Enjoy!

NUTRIENT FACTS	TOTAL	PER SERVING
Calories (kCal):	334	37.11
Proteins (g):	10	1.11
Carbohydrates (g):	26	2.89
Fats (g):	23	2.56
Potassium (mg):	3398	377.56
Phosphorus (mg):	860	95.56
Sodium (mg):	3002	333.67

CHEESY TORTILLA ROLLUPS

Servings:	4	Preparation Time	10 mins

INGREDIENTS

½ cup whipped cream cheese
2 flour tortillas, burrito size
½ cup raw spinach leaves, chopped
2 tablespoons onion, diced
2 tablespoons pimento, diced
½ cup crushed pineapple, drained
3 ounces unprocessed cooked turkey breast, diced small
1 teaspoon Mrs. Dash® original blend herb seasoning

DIRECTIONS

1. First, place cream cheese over each tortilla to cover and sprinkle with Mrs. Dash® herb seasoning.
2. In a bowl, put remaining ingredients and mix.
3. Divide mixed ingredients into 2 portions and place half on each tortillas.
4. Roll it up and slice each roll into 4 pieces.

NUTRIENT FACTS

	TOTAL	PER SERVING
Calories (kCal):	956	239
Proteins (g):	41.3	10.33
Carbohydrates (g):	99.5	24.88
Fats (g):	45.67	11.42
Potassium (mg):	1080	270
Phosphorus (mg):	415	103.75
Sodium (mg):	916	229

Hydration Tips and Safe Beverages

Hydration is essential for everyone, including individuals with chronic kidney disease (CKD). However, those with CKD may need to monitor and potentially limit their fluid intake, particularly as the disease progresses. Here are some key hydration tips and safe beverage suggestions to consider:

Monitor Your Fluid Intake

Depending on the stage of your CKD and whether you're on dialysis, your healthcare provider or dietitian may recommend limiting your fluid intake. This includes not only drinks but also foods that are liquid at room temperature, such as ice cream or gelatin.

Choose Water

Water is typically the best choice for hydration. It is calorie-free and free from sodium, potassium, and phosphorus, making it an ideal option for maintaining hydration without adding unnecessary nutrients that could affect kidney health.

Limit High-Potassium Drinks

Avoid beverages that are high in potassium, such as:

- Orange juice
- Tomato juice
- Prune juice
- Certain sports drinks

Limit High-Phosphorus Drinks

Stay away from drinks that are high in phosphorus, including:

- Beer
- Cola drinks

Many dark-colored sodas contain phosphorus additives that can contribute to elevated phosphorus levels in the body.

Limit Sodium-Rich Drinks

Be cautious with beverages that may be high in sodium, such as:

- Canned soups and broths
- Bottled sauces
- Sports drinks
- Any drinks labeled as "high in sodium"

Limit Alcohol

Alcohol can lead to dehydration and place additional stress on your kidneys. It's best to limit or avoid alcohol consumption altogether.

Beware of Coffee and Tea

Both coffee and tea can be high in potassium. If you choose to drink them, limit your intake to small amounts and consider counting them towards your daily fluid allowance.

Avoid Energy Drinks

Energy drinks often contain high levels of sodium, sugar, and caffeine, which can be detrimental to your kidney health.

Herbal Infusions

Some herbal teas may be a suitable option, but it's crucial to check with your healthcare provider or dietitian first, as certain herbs can affect kidney function.

Stay Cool

Try to avoid overheating, as sweating leads to increased water loss. Staying cool can help you maintain proper hydration levels.

Final Reminder

These guidelines are general in nature, and individual hydration needs can vary significantly. Always consult with your healthcare provider or dietitian to determine the best hydration plan tailored to your specific situation.

Part III: The Complete Kidney-Friendly Food Reference

Chapter 7: The Renal Diet Food List

Welcome to the heart of this book! As previously mentioned, the data contained in this food list has been meticulously curated by a dedicated team of dietitians and nephrology nurses. They have invested countless hours gathering scientific data from reputable sources, including the USDA Food Data Central, ensuring that this information is accurate and reliable for your chronic kidney disease (CKD) diet management as prescribed by your physician and dietitian. For your convenience, you can also find an index in Appendix C (page 170) to quickly locate specific foods.

How to Use the Charts

Navigating the food list is simple! Here's a step-by-step guide to help you utilize the charts effectively:

1. Categorization: The charts are organized into general food groups:

    - Carbohydrates
    - Fats (oils, nuts, and seeds)
    - Milk
    - Fruits & Vegetables
    - Vegetable Proteins
    - Meats, Poultry, & Seafood
    - Herbs & Spices

2. Finding Specific Foods: Locate your desired food item through the categories or use the indices available in Appendix C (page 175).

3. Standardized Measurements: Each food group is further categorized by preparation styles, standardized to a measurement of 100 grams. Below this, you will find additional measurements (slices, teaspoons, tablespoons, or cups) along with their corresponding weights in grams.

4. Nutrient Information: For each 100 grams of food, you will find the corresponding amounts of essential nutrients, including:

- Calories
- Carbohydrates
- Proteins
- Fats
- Sodium
- Phosphorus
- Potassium

5. Calculating Nutrient Content: You can divide or multiply the nutrient values based on the amount of food you are preparing in your recipe.

Example 1: Actual Nutrient Content in Your Recipe

ASPARAGUS	SERVING QUANTITY	SERVING UNIT	CALORIES (kCal)	PROTEIN (g)	TOTAL CARBOHYDRATES (g)	SODIUM (mg)	POTASSIUM (mg)	PHOSPHORUS (mg)	TOTAL FAT (g)
boiled,	100.00	g	22	2.4	4.1	14.00	224.00	54.00	0.22
drained	90.00	g	20	2.2	3.7	12.60	201.60	48.60	0.20
	0.50	c							

Let's say your recipe calls for 1 cup of boiled asparagus. According to the food list chart, 90 grams of boiled asparagus is equivalent to ½ cup. Since you need a full cup, you would multiply the nutrient values by 2.

For 1 cup of asparagus, the nutrient content would be:

- Calories: 40 kCal
- Protein: 4.4 g
- Carbohydrates: 7.4 g
- Fats: 0.40 g
- Sodium: 25.2 mg
- Potassium: 403 mg
- Phosphorus: 97.2 mg

Example 2: More on Reading and Using the Chart

ASPARAGUS	SERVING QUANTITY	SERVING UNIT	CALORIES (kcal)	PROTEIN (g)	TOTAL CARBOHYDRATES (g)	SODIUM (mg)	POTASSIUM (mg)	PHOSPHORUS (mg)	TOTAL FAT (g)
boiled,	100.00	g	22	2.4	4.1	14.00	224.00	54.00	0.22
drained	90.00	g	20	2.2	3.7	12.60	201.60	48.60	0.20
	0.50	c							
frozen	100.00	g	24	3.2	4.1	8.00	253.00	64.00	0.23
	87.00	g	21	2.8	3.6	6.96	220.11	55.68	0.20
	6.00	pcs							

Consider 6 pieces of frozen asparagus, which weigh approximately 87 grams. You would reference the nutrient values based on the 87-gram line. If you wish to reduce your potassium intake, you might choose to eat only 3 pieces, which would lower the potassium content from 220.11 mg to approximately 110 mg.

Alternatively, using a kitchen scale to measure your food allows you to adjust your intake based on the 100-gram standard, tailoring your consumption to meet your daily needs and restrictions effectively.

A. Vegetable Proteins

Hey there!

Do you need to print out this Food List?

You can download a printable version of this chart by scanning the QR code below or copying the link on your computer browser.

https://go.renaltracker.com/printfoodlist

BEANS

BEANS	SERVING QUANTITY	SERVING UNIT	CALORIES (kCal)	PROTEIN (g)	TOTAL CARBOHYDRATES (g)	SODIUM (mg)	POTASSIUM (mg)	PHOSPHORUS (mg)	TOTAL FAT (g)
Lentils/Pinto/N	100.00	g	131	8.6	23.9	1.67	398.91	165.76	0.49
avy	92.00	g	121	8.0	22.0	1.54	367.00	152.50	0.45
	0.50	c							
Lima	100.00	g	113	6.8	20.2	8.00	467.00	136.00	0.86
	78.00	g	88	5.3	15.7	6.24	364.26	106.08	0.67
	0.50	c							
Broad or Fava	100.00	g	72	5.6	11.7	50.00	250.00	95.00	0.60
	81.75	g	59	4.6	9.6	40.88	204.38	77.66	0.49
	0.75	c							
Black beans,	100.00	g	132	8.9	23.7	1.00	355.00	140.00	0.54
boiled	86.00	g	114	7.6	20.4	0.86	305.30	120.40	0.46
	0.50	c							
Mungo, boiled	100.00	g	105	7.5	18.3	7.00	231.00	156.00	0.55
	90.00	g	95	6.8	16.5	6.30	207.90	140.40	0.50
	0.50	c							
sprouts, Mung	100.00	g	30	3.0	5.9	6.00	149.00	54.00	0.18
	78.00	g	23	2.4	4.6	4.68	116.22	42.12	0.14
	0.75	c							
Kidney, boiled	100.00	g	127	8.7	22.8	1.00	405.00	138.00	0.50
	88.50	g	112	7.7	20.2	0.89	358.43	122.13	0.44
	0.50	c							
Navy, boiled	100.00	g	140	8.2	26.1	0.00	389.00	144.00	0.62
	91.00	g	127	7.5	23.7	0.00	353.99	131.04	0.56
	0.50	c							
Lupin, boiled	100.00	g	119	15.6	9.9	4.00	245.00	128.00	2.92
	83.00	g	99	12.9	8.2	3.32	203.35	106.24	2.42
	0.50	c							
Pinto, frozen	100.00	g	170	9.8	32.5	92.00	755.98	117.00	0.50
	94.49	g	161	9.3	31.0	86.93	714.34	110.55	0.47
	3.33	oz							
Pinto, boiled	100.00	g	143	9.0	26.2	1.00	436.00	147.00	0.65
	85.50	g	122	7.7	22.4	0.86	372.78	125.69	0.56
	0.50	c							
White (Cannellini),	100.00	g	139	9.7	25.1	6.00	561.00	113.00	0.35
boiled no salt	89.50	g	124	8.7	22.5	5.37	502.10	101.14	0.31
	0.50	c							

BEANS

	SERVING QUANTITY	SERVING UNIT	CALORIES (kcal)	PROTEIN (g)	TOTAL CARBOHYDRATES (g)	SODIUM (mg)	POTASSIUM (mg)	PHOSPHORUS (mg)	TOTAL FAT (g)
White, small,	100.00	g	142	9.0	25.8	2.00	463.00	169.00	0.64
boiled, no salt	89.50	g	127	8.0	23.1	1.79	414.39	151.26	0.57
	0.50	c							
sprouts, Kidney	100.00	g	29	4.2	4.1	6.00	187.00	37.00	0.50
	92.00	g	27	3.9	3.8	5.52	172.04	34.04	0.46
	0.50	c							
sprouts, Navy	100.00	g	67	6.2	13.1	13.00	307.00	100.00	0.70
	78.00	g	52	4.8	10.2	10.14	239.46	78.00	0.55
	0.75	c							
sprouts, Pinto	100.00	g	62	5.3	11.6	153.0	307.00	94.00	0.90
	85.05	g	53	4.5	9.9	130.1	262.10	79.95	0.77
	3.00	oz							
French, boiled	100.00	g	129	7.1	24.0	6.00	370.00	102.00	0.76
	88.50	g	114	6.2	21.3	5.31	327.45	90.27	0.67
	0.50	c							
baked, prepared	100.00	g	155	5.5	21.6	422.0	358.00	109.00	5.15
	126.50	g	196	7.0	27.4	533.8	452.87	138.00	6.51
	0.50	c							
Refried, canned	100.00	g	90	5.0	13.6	370.0	319.00	92.00	2.01
	119.00	g	107	5.9	16.1	440.3	379.61	109.48	2.39
	0.50	c							

CHICKPEAS

	SERVING QUANTITY	SERVING UNIT	CALORIES (kcal)	PROTEIN (g)	TOTAL CARBOHYDRATES (g)	SODIUM (mg)	POTASSIUM (mg)	PHOSPHORUS (mg)	TOTAL FAT (g)
garbanzos/ bengal gram, canned	100.00	g	88	4.9	13.5	278.0	144.00	80.00	1.95
	120.00	g	106	5.9	16.2	333.6	172.80	96.00	2.34
	0.50	c							
garbanzos/ bengal gram, boiled	100.00	g	164	8.9	27.4	7.00	291.00	168.00	2.59
	82.00	g	134	7.3	22.5	5.74	238.62	137.76	2.12
	0.50	c							
garbanzos/ bengal gram, canned drained, rinsed in tap water	100.00	g	138	7.0	22.9	212.0	109.00	80.00	2.47
	152.00	g	210	10.7	34.8	322.3	165.68	121.60	3.75
	1.00	c							
garbanzos/ bengal gram, canned low sodium	100	g	88	4.9	13.5	132.0	144.00	80.00	1.95
	240	g	211	11.8	32.4	316.8	345.60	192.00	4.68
	1	c							
flour	100.00	g	387	22.4	57.8	64.00	846.00	318.00	6.69
	92.00	g	110	6.4	16.4	18.14	239.84	90.15	1.90
	1.00	c							

TOFU

	SERVING QUANTITY	SERVING UNIT	CALORIES (kCal)	PROTEIN (g)	TOTAL CARBOHYDRATES (g)	SODIUM (mg)	POTASSIUM (mg)	PHOSPHORUS (mg)	TOTAL FAT (g)
soft with calcium sulfate and magnesium chloride (Nigari)	100.00	g	61	7.2	1.2	8.00	120.00	92.00	3.69
	85.05	g	52	6.1	1.0	6.80	102.06	78.25	3.14
	3.00	oz							
firm with calcium sulfate and magnesium chloride (Nigari)	100.00	g	78	9.0	2.9	12.00	148.00	121.00	4.17
	85.05	g	66	7.7	2.4	10.21	125.87	102.91	3.55
	3.00	oz							
silken tofu (Vitasoy USA)	100.00	g	43	4.8	0.6	2.00	na	na	2.40
	91.00	g	39	4.4	0.5	1.82	na	na	2.18
	0.20	package							

TEMPEH

	SERVING QUANTITY	SERVING UNIT	CALORIES (kCal)	PROTEIN (g)	TOTAL CARBOHYDRATES (g)	SODIUM (mg)	POTASSIUM (mg)	PHOSPHORUS (mg)	TOTAL FAT (g)
raw	100.00	g	192	20.3	7.6	9.00	412.0	266.0	10.80
	83.00	g	159	16.8	6.3	7.47	341.9	220.8	8.96
	0.50	c							
cooked	100.00	g	185	19.9	7.6	14.00	401.0	253.0	11.38

EDAMAME

	SERVING QUANTITY	SERVING UNIT	CALORIES (kCal)	PROTEIN (g)	TOTAL CARBOHYDRATES (g)	SODIUM (mg)	POTASSIUM (mg)	PHOSPHORUS (mg)	TOTAL FAT (g)
frozen, unprepared	100.00	g	109	11.2	7.6	6.00	482.0	161.0	4.73
	118.00	g	129	13.2	9.0	7.08	568.7	189.9	5.58
	1.00	c							
frozen, prepared	100.00	g	121	11.9	8.9	6.00	436.0	261.9	5.20
	155.00	g	188	18.5	13.8	9.30	676	169	8.06
	1.00	c							

SPIRULINA

	SERVING QUANTITY	SERVING UNIT	CALORIES (kCal)	PROTEIN (g)	TOTAL CARBOHYDRATES (g)	SODIUM (mg)	POTASSIUM (mg)	PHOSPHORUS (mg)	TOTAL FAT (g)
seaweed, fresh/raw	100.00	g	26	5.9	2.4	98.00	127	11.00	0.39
	28.35	g	7	1.7	0.7	27.78	36.00	3.12	0.11
	1.00	oz							
seaweed, dried	100.00	g	290	57.5	23.9	1,048	1363	118	7.72
	112.00	g	325	64.4	26.8	1,174	1527	133	8.65
	1.00	c							

B. Animal Protein

(Meats, Poultry, and Seafood)

Hey there!

Do you need to print out this Food List?

You can download a printable version of this chart by scanning the QR code below or copying the link on your computer browser.

https://go.renaltracker.com/printfoodlist

CHICKEN	SERVING QUANTITY	SERVING UNIT	CALORIES (kCal)	PROTEIN (g)	TOTAL CARBOHYDRATES (g)	SODIUM (mg)	POTASSIUM (mg)	PHOSPHORUS (mg)	TOTAL FAT (g)
ground, raw	100.00	g	143	17.4	0.0	60.00	522.00	178.00	8.10
meat and skin,	100.00	g	215	18.6	0.0	70.00	189.00	147.00	15.06
raw	113.40	g	244	21.1	0.0	79.38	214.33	166.70	17.08
	4.00	oz							
meat and skin,	100.00	g	239	27.3	0.0	82.00	223.00	182.00	13.60
roasted	85.05	g	203	23.2	0.0	69.74	189.66	154.79	11.57
	3.00	oz							
thigh meat only,	100.00	g	218	28.2	1.2	95.00	259.00	199.00	10.30
fried	85.05	g	185	24.0	1.0	80.80	220.28	169.25	8.76
	3.00	oz							
thigh meat only,	100.00	g	179	24.8	0.0	106.00	269.00	230.00	8.15
roasted	85.05	g	152	21.1	0.0	90.15	228.78	195.61	6.93
	3.00	oz							
wing meat only,	100.00	g	211	30.2	0.0	91.00	208.00	164.00	9.15
fried	85.05	g	179	25.6	0.0	77.39	176.90	139.48	7.78
	3.00	oz							
wing meat only,	100.00	g	203	30.5	0.0	92.00	210.00	166.00	8.13
roasted	85.05	g	173	26.0	0.0	78.25	178.60	141.18	6.91
	3.00	oz							
wing meat only,	100.00	g	181	27.2	0.0	73.00	153.00	134.00	7.18
stewed	85.05	g	154	23.1	0.0	62.09	130.12	113.97	6.11
	3.00	oz							
back meat only,	100.00	g	288	30.0	5.7	99.00	251.00	176.00	4.12
fried	85.05	g	245	25.5	4.8	84.20	213.47	149.69	3.50
	3.00	oz							
back meat only,	100.00	g	239	28.2	0.0	96.00	237.00	165.00	13.16
roasted	85.05	g	203	24.0	0.0	81.65	201.57	140.33	11.19
	3.00	oz							
back meat only,	100.00	g	209	25.3	0.0	67.00	158.00	130.00	11.19
stewed	85.05	g	178	21.5	0.0	56.98	134.38	110.56	9.52
	3.00	oz							
drumstick meat	100.00	g	195	28.6	0.0	96.00	249.00	186.00	8.08
only, fried	85.05	g	166	24.3	0.0	81.65	211.77	158.19	6.87
	3.00	oz							
drumstick meat	100.00	g	155	24.2	0.0	128.00	256.00	200.00	5.70
only, roasted	85.05	g	132	20.6	0.0	108.86	217.73	170.10	4.85
	3	oz							

CHICKEN

	SERVING QUANTITY	SERVING UNIT	CALORIES (kcal)	PROTEIN (g)	TOTAL CARBOHYDRATES (g)	SODIUM (mg)	POTASSIUM (mg)	PHOSPHORUS (mg)	TOTAL FAT (g)
drumstick meat only, stewed	100.00	g	169	27.5	0.0	80.00	199.00	150.00	5.71
	85.05 3.00	g oz	144	23.4	0.0	68.04	169.25	127.57	4.86
leg meat only, fried	100.00	g	208	28.4	0.7	96.00	254.00	193.00	9.32
	85.05 3.00	g oz	177	24.1	0.6	81.65	216.02	164.14	7.93
leg meat only, roasted	100.00	g	174	24.2	0.0	99.00	269.00	205.00	7.80
	85.05 3.00	g oz	148	20.6	0.0	84.20	228.78	174.35	6.63
leg meat only, stewed	100.00	g	185	26.3	0.0	78.00	190.00	149.00	8.06
	85.05 3.00	g oz	157	22.3	0.0	66.34	161.59	126.72	6.85
pate, chicken liver, canned	100.00	g	201	13.5	6.6	386.0	95.00	175.00	13.10
	52.00 4.00	g tbsp	105	7.0	3.4	200.7	49.40	91.00	6.81
chicken tenders, fast food	100.00	g	271	19.2	17.3	769.0	373.00	282.00	13.95
	62.00 4.00	g pcs	168	11.9	10.7	476.8	231.26	174.84	8.65
chicken patty, frozen, cooked	100.00	g	287	14.9	12.8	532.0	261.00	208.00	19.58
bratwurst, chicken, cooked	100.00	g	176	19.4	0.0	72.00	211.00	160.00	10.30
	83.92 2.96	g oz	148	16.3	0.0	60.42	177.06	134.27	8.69
sausage, chicken/beef, smoked	100.00	g	295	18.5	0.0	1,020	139.00	111.00	244.0(
	138.00 1.00	g c	251	15.7	0.0	867.5	118.22	94.41	20.41

TURKEY

TURKEY	SERVING QUANTITY	SERVING UNIT	CALORIES (kcal)	PROTEIN (g)	TOTAL CARBOHYDRATES (g)	SODIUM (mg)	POTASSIUM (mg)	PHOSPHORUS (mg)	TOTAL FAT (g)
breast, meat & skin, raw	100.00	g	144	21.6	0.1	112.00	224.00	183.00	5.64
	113.40	g	163	24.5	0.2	127.01	254.02	207.52	6.40
	4.00	oz							
breast, meat & skin, roasted	100.00	g	189	28.6	0.1	103.00	239.00	223.00	7.39
	85.05	g	161	24.3	0.1	87.60	203.27	189.66	6.29
	3.00	oz							
breast, meat only, raw	100.00	g	114	23.3	0.0	74.00	267.00	185.00	2.33
	85.05	g	97	19.9	0.0	62.94	227.08	157.34	1.98
	3.00	oz							
breast, meat only, roasted	100.00	g	136	29.5	0.0	114.00	297.00	253.00	1.97
	85.05	g	116	25.1	0.0	96.96	252.60	215.17	1.68
	3.00	oz							
ground, raw	100.00	g	148	20.0	0.0	58.00	237.00	200.00	7.66
	113.40	g	168	22.3	0.0	65.77	268.76	226.80	8.69
	4.00	oz							
ground, cooked	100.00	g	203	27.4	0.0	78.00	294.00	254.00	10.40
	85.05	g	173	23.3	0.0	66.34	250.04	216.02	8.85
	3.00	oz							
white rotisserie, deli cut	100.00	g	112	13.5	7.7	1,200	349.00	158.00	3.00
	56.70	g	64	7.7	4.4	680.40	197.88	89.59	1.70
	2.00	oz							
ham, extra lean, sliced	100.00	g	134	19.6	0.9	1,038	299.00	304.00	5.80
	20.00	g	27	3.9	0.2	207.60	59.80	60.80	1.16
	1.00	pc							
pastrami, sliced	100.00	g	139	16.3	3.3	1,123	345.00	200.00	6.21
	56.70	g	79	9.2	1.9	636.74	195.62	113.40	3.52
	2.00	slices							
bologna	100.00	g	209	11.4	4.7	1,071	135.00	114.00	16.05
	56.70	g	119	6.5	2.7	607.26	76.55	64.64	9.10
	2.00	slices							
salami	100.00	g	172	19.2	1.6	1,107	216.00	266.00	9.21
	56.70	g	98	10.9	0.9	627.67	122.47	150.82	5.22
	2.00	slices							
bacon, turkey, cooked	100.00	g	382	29.6	3.1	2,285	395.00	460.00	27.90
	28.35	g	108	8.4	0.9	647.80	111.98	130.41	7.91
	1.00	oz							
bacon, turkey, low sodium	100.00	g	253	13.3	4.8	900.00	156.00	145.00	20.00
	15.00	g	38	2.0	0.7	135.00	23.40	21.75	3.00
	1.00	svg							
sausage, turkey, cooked	100.00	g	196	23.9	0.0	665.00	298.00	202.00	10.44
	56.70	g	111	13.6	0.0	377.06	168.97	114.53	5.92
	2.00	oz							

EGG

	SERVING QUANTITY	SERVING UNIT	CALORIES (Kcal)	PROTEIN (g)	TOTAL CARBOHYDRATES (g)	SODIUM (mg)	POTASSIUM (mg)	PHOSPHORUS (mg)	TOTAL FAT (g)
chicken, raw, large	100.00	g	143	12.6	0.7	142.00	138.00	198.00	9.51
	50.00	g	72	6.3	0.4	71.00	69.00	99.00	4.76
	1.00	pc							
chicken, fried, large	100.00	g	196	13.6	0.8	207.00	152.00	215.00	14.84
	46.00	g	90	6.3	0.4	95.22	69.92	98.90	6.83
	1.00	pc							
chicken, poached, large	100.00	g	143	12.5	0.7	297.00	138.00	197.00	9.47
	50.00	g	72	6.3	0.4	148.50	69.00	98.50	4.74
	1.00	pc							
chicken, hard boiled, large	100.00	g	155	12.6	1.1	124.00	126.00	172.00	10.61
	50.00	g	78	6.3	0.6	62.00	63.00	86.00	5.31
	1.00	pc							
scrambled, fast food	100.00	g	212	13.8	2.1	187.00	147.00	242.00	16.18
	94.00	g	199	13.0	2.0	175.78	138.18	227.48	15.21
	2.00	pc							
substitute, liquid	100.00	g	84	12.0	0.6	177.00	330.00	121.00	3.31
	251.00	g	211	30.1	1.6	444.27	828.30	303.71	8.31
	1.00	c							
substitute, powder	100.00	g	443	55.8	22	798.19	742.31	476.92	12.97
	9.92	g	44	5.5	2.2	79.20	73.66	47.32	1.29
	0.35	oz							
substitute, frozen	100.00	g	160	11.3	3.2	199.00	213.00	72.00	11.11
	60.00	g	96	6.8	1.9	119.40	127.80	43.20	6.67
	0.25	c							
chicken, egg whites only, raw large egg	100.00	g	52	10.9	0.7	166.00	163.00	15.00	0.17
	33.00	g	17	3.6	0.2	54.78	53.79	4.95	0.06
	1.00	pc							
chicken, yolk only, raw large egg	100.00	g	322	15.9	3.6	48.00	109.00	390.00	26.54
	17.00	g	55	2.7	0.6	8.16	18.53	66.30	4.51
	1.00	pc							
chicken, whole, raw, frozen	100.00	g	147	12.3	1.0	128.00	135.00	193.00	9.95
	56.70	g	83	7.0	0.6	72.57	76.54	109.43	5.64
	2.00	oz							
yolk only, frozen, raw	100.00	g	296	15.5	0.8	67.00	121.00	419.99	25.60
	56.70	g	168	8.8	0.5	37.99	68.61	238.14	14.51
	2.00	oz							
whites, frozen, raw	100.00	g	48	10.2	1.0	169.00	169.00	13.00	0.00
	56.70	g	27	5.8	0.6	95.82	95.82	7.37	0.00
	2.00	oz							
duck, raw	100.00	g	185	12.8	1.5	146.00	222.00	220.00	13.77
	70.00	g	130	9.0	1.0	102.20	155.40	154.00	9.64
	1.00	pc							
quail, raw	100.00	g	158	13.1	0.4	141.00	132.00	226.00	11.09
	9.00	g	14	1.2	0.0	12.69	11.88	20.34	1.00
	1.00	pc							

PORK

PORK	SERVING QUANTITY	SERVING UNIT	CALORIES (kcal)	PROTEIN (g)	TOTAL CARBOHYDRATES (g)	SODIUM (mg)	POTASSIUM (mg)	PHOSPHORUS (mg)	TOTAL FAT (g)
ground, cooked	100.00	g	297	25.7	0.0	73.00	362.00	226.00	20.77
	85.05	g	253	21.9	0.0	62.09	307.88	192.21	17.66
	3.00	oz							
ground, raw	100.00	g	263	16.9	0.0	56.00	287.00	175.00	21.19
	113.40	g	298	19.1	0.0	63.50	325.46	198.45	24.03
	4.00	oz							
loin, sirloin, roasts, *separable lean roasted*	100.00	g	204	27.8	0.0	59.00	352.00	235.00	9.44
	85.05	g	174	23.6	0.0	50.18	299.37	199.87	8.03
	3.00	oz							
loin, center rib, separable lean, roasted	100.00	g	206	28.8	0.0	95.00	287.00	244.00	9.21
	85.05	g	175	24.5	0.0	80.80	244.09	207.52	7.83
	3.00	oz							
loin, sirloin, *boneless, separable lean roasted*	100.00	g	178	30.4	0.0	66.00	408.00	311.00	5.31
	85.05	g	151	25.9	0.0	56.13	347.00	264.50	4.52
	3.00	oz							
loin, center rib, *boneless roasted*	100.00	g	214	28.8	0.0	50.00	363.00	222.00	10.13
	85.05	g	182	24.5	0.0	42.52	308.73	188.81	8.62
	3.00	oz							
shoulder blade, *boston roasts roasted* turkey, salt.	100.00	g	232	24.2	0.0	88.00	427.00	235.00	14.30
	85.05	g	197	20.6	0.0	74.84	363.16	199.87	12.16
	3.00	oz							
shoulder, whole, roasted	100.00	g	230	25.3	0.0	74.96	345.80	220.87	13.53
	85.05	g	196	21.5	0.0	63.75	294.10	187.85	11.51
	3.00	oz							
loin, whole, roasted	100.00	g	209	28.6	0.0	58.00	425.00	249.00	9.63
	85.05	g	178	24.3	0.0	49.33	361.46	211.77	8.19
	3.00	oz							
leg or ham, whole, roasted	100.00	g	211	29.4	0.0	64.00	373.00	281.00	9.44
	85.05	g	179	25.0	0.0	54.43	317.23	238.99	8.03
	3.00	oz							
loin, tenderloin, *separable lean & fat roasted*	100.00	g	147	26.0	0.0	57.00	419.00	265.00	3.96
	85.05	g	125	22.2	0.0	48.48	356.36	225.38	3.37
	3.00	oz							
ground, cooked	100.00	g	297	25.7	0.0	73.00	362.00	226.00	20.77
	85.05	g	253	21.9	0.0	62.09	307.88	192.21	17.66
	3.00	oz							

PORK

	SERVING QUANTITY	SERVING UNIT	CALORIES (kCal)	PROTEIN (g)	TOTAL CARBOHYDRATES (g)	SODIUM (mg)	POTASSIUM (mg)	PHOSPHORUS (mg)	TOTAL FAT (g)
bacon, cured, broiled, panfried or roasted	100.00	g	541	37.0	1.4	1,717.0	565.0	533.0	41.78
	8.00	g	43	3.0	0.1	137.36	45.20	42.64	3.34
	1.00	slice							
bacon, reduced sodium, cured broiled, panfried or roasted	100.00	g	541	37.0	1.4	1,030.0	565.0	533.0	41.78
	56.70	g	307	21.0	0.8	584.01	320.4	302.2	23.69
	2.00	oz							
country style ribs, separable lean & fat roasted	100.00	g	359	21.8	0.0	52.00	322.0	214.0	29.46
	85.05	g	305	18.5	0.0	44.23	273.9	182.0	25.06
	3.00	oz							
sirloin, chops or roasts, boneless, raw	100.00	g	121	22.8	0.0	63.00	354.0	251.0	2.59
	113.40	g	137	25.9	0.0	71.44	401.4	284.6	2.94
	4.00	oz							
kidney, braised	100.00	g	151	25.4	0.0	80.00	143.0	240.0	4.70
	85.05	g	128	21.6	0.0	68.04	121.6	204.1	4.00
	3.00	oz							
liver, braised	100.00	g	165	26.0	3.8	49.00	150.0	241.0	4.40
	85.05	g	140	22.1	3.2	41.67	127.6	205.0	3.74
	3.00	oz							
ham, minced, sliced	100.00	g	263	16.3	1.8	1,245.0	311.0	157.0	20.68
	21.00	g	55	3.4	0.4	261.45	65.31	32.97	4.34
	1.00	slice							
ham, extra lean, 5% fat	100.00	g	107	16.9	0.7	944.99	463.0	252.0	4.04
	85.05	g	91	14.3	0.6	803.71	393.8	214.3	3.44
	3.00	oz							
ham, low sodium, cured, cooked	100.00	g	165	22.0	0.5	969.00	362.0	248.0	7.70
	85.05	g	140	18.7	0.4	824.13	307.9	210.9	6.55
	3.00	oz							
sausages, Kielbasa, grilled	100.00	g	337	12.5	5.0	1,062	306.0	204.0	29.68
	85.05	g	287	10.6	4.3	903.22	260.3	173.5	25.24
	3.00	oz							
Kielbasa, panfried	100.00	g	333	12.4	4.8	1,046	304.0	199.0	29.43
	85.05	g	283	10.5	4.1	889.61	258.6	169.3	25.03
	3.00	oz							
Beerwurst, pork/beef	100.00	g	276	14.0	4.3	732.00	244.0	135.0	22.53
	56.70	g	156	7.9	2.4	415.04	138.4	76.6	12.77
	2.00	oz							

PORK

	SERVING QUANTITY	SERVING UNIT	CALORIES (Kcal)	PROTEIN (g)	TOTAL CARBOHYDRATES (g)	SODIUM (mg)	POTASSIUM (mg)	PHOSPHORUS (mg)	TOTAL FAT (g)
Italian Sweet, links	100	g	149	16.1	2.1	570.00	194.00	103.00	8.42
	85.05 3	g oz	127	13.7	1.8	484.79	165.00	87.60	7.16
Polish, pork, cooked	100	g	326	14.1	1.6	875.99	237.00	136.00	28.72
	56.70 2	g oz	185	8.0	0.9	496.68	134.38	77.11	16.28
Bratwurst, pork, cooked	100	g	333	13.7	2.9	845.99	347.99	208.00	29.18
	56.70 2	g oz	189	7.8	1.6	479.67	197.31	117.93	16.54
meatloaf/ luncheon meat pork/beef	100	g	260	15.4	1.6	1,182	245.00	122.00	20.90
	2 1	g slice	60	3.5	0.4	271.86	56.35	28.06	4.81
peperoni, beef/pork	100	g	504	19.3	1.2	1,582	274.00	158.00	46.28
	56.70 2	g oz	286	11.0	0.7	896.98	155.36	89.58	26.24
salami, italian, pork	100	g	425	21.7	1.2	1,890	340.00	229.00	37.00
	28.35 1	g oz	120	6.2	0.3	535.82	96.39	64.92	10.49

BEEF	SERVING QUANTITY	SERVING UNIT	CALORIES (Kcal)	PROTEIN (g)	TOTAL CARBOHYDRATES (g)	SODIUM (mg)	POTASSIUM (mg)	PHOSPHORUS (mg)	TOTAL FAT (g)
chuck eyeroast, boneless, all grades o" fat, separable lean only, **roasted**	3 85.05 3.00	g g oz	183 156	26.7 22.7	0.0 0.0	68.04 80.00	344.00 292.57	210.00 178.61	8.46 7.20
chuck eyeroast, boneless, all grades separable lean only, o", **raw**	100.00 85.05 3.00	g g oz	137 117	20.6 17.5	0.0 0.0	85.00 72.29	357.00 303.63	204.00 173.50	6.01 5.11
chuck eyeroast, boneless, all grades sep lean & fat, o" fat, **roasted**	100.00 85.05 3.00	g g oz	236 201	24.6 21.0	0.0 0.0	76.00 64.64	308.00 261.95	187.00 159.04	15.29 13.00
chuck eyeroast, boneless, all grades sep lean & fat, o" fat, **raw**	100.00 85.05 3.00	g g oz	173 147	19.3 16.4	0.0 0.0	82.00 69.74	367.00 312.13	187.00 159.04	10.67 9.07
jerky	100.00 28.35 1.00	g g oz	410 116	33.2 9.4	11 3.1	1,785 506.05	597.00 169.25	407.00 115.38	25.60 7.26
corned beef, brisket, **raw**	100.00 113.40 4.00	g g oz	198 225	14.7 16.7	0.1 0.2	1,217 1,380	297.00 336.80	117.00 132.68	14.90 16.90
corned beef, brisket, **cooked**	100.00 85.05 3.00	g g oz	251 213	18.2 15.5	0.5 0.4	927.99 827.53	145.00 123.32	125.00 106.31	18.98 16.14
broth cube 1 cube, 6 fl. oz prepared	100.00 3.60 1.00	g g cube	170 6	17.3 0.6	16 0.6	24,000 864.00	403.00 14.51	225.00 8.10	4.00 0.14
liver, pan fried	100.00 81.00 1.00	g g slice	175 142	26.5 21.5	5.2 4.2	77.00 62.37	351.00 284.31	485.00 392.85	4.68 3.79
liver, braised	100.00 85.05 3.00	g g oz	191 162	29.1 24.7	5.1 4.4	79.00 67.19	352.00 299.37	496.99 422.69	5.26 4.47
tongue, simmered	100.00 85.05 3.00	g g oz	284 242	19.3 16.4	0.0 0.0	65.00 55.28	184.00 156.49	145.00 123.32	22.30 18.97
kidney simmered	100.00 85.05 3.00	g g oz	158 134	27.3 23.2	0.0 0.0	94.00 79.95	135.00 114.82	304.00 258.55	4.65 3.95
tripe, simmered	100.00 85.05 3.00	g g oz	94 80	11.7 10.0	2.0 1.7	68.00 57.83	42.00 35.72	66.00 56.13	4.05 3.44

LAMB

	SERVING QUANTITY	SERVING UNIT	CALORIES (kcal)	PROTEIN (g)	TOTAL CARBOHYDRATES (g)	SODIUM (mg)	POTASSIUM (mg)	PHOSPHORUS (mg)	TOTAL FAT (g)
tenderloin, New Zealand, separable lean only, raw	100.00	g	116	20.5	0.0	49.00	381.00	222.00	3.81
	85.05	g	99	17.5	0.0	41.67	324.04	188.81	3.24
	3.00	oz							
loin, NZ, separable lean, frozen, broiled	100.00	g	199	29.3	0.0	55.00	189.00	240.00	8.24
	85.05	g	169	24.9	0.0	46.78	160.74	204.12	7.01
	3.00	oz							
australian, separable lean, 1/8" fat, cooked	100.00	g	201	26.7	0.0	80.00	318.00	207.00	9.63
	85.05	g	171	22.7	0.0	68.04	270.46	176.05	8.19
	3.00	oz							
Australian, separable lean, 1/8" fat, raw	100.00	g	142	20.3	0.0	83.00	320.00	188.00	6.18
	113.40	g	161	23.0	0.0	94.12	362.88	213.19	7.01
	4.00	oz							
Australian, ground, 85%Lean/15%fat, raw	100.00	g	255	17.1	0.0	65.49	na	na	20.17
	85.05	g	217	14.6	0.0	77.00	na	na	17.61
	3.00	oz							
NZ, rib, separable lean, frozen, raw	100.00	g	160	20.7	0.0	67.00	309.00	185.00	8.61
	113.40	g	181	23.4	0.0	75.98	350.41	209.79	9.76
	4.00	oz							
NZ, rib, separable lean, frozen, roasted	100.00	g	193	24.4	0.0	72.00	323.00	209.00	10.63
	85.05	g	164	20.8	0.0	61.24	274.71	177.75	9.04
	3.00	oz							

VEAL

	SERVING QUANTITY	SERVING UNIT	CALORIES (kcal)	PROTEIN (g)	TOTAL CARBOHYDRATES (g)	SODIUM (mg)	POTASSIUM (mg)	PHOSPHORUS (mg)	TOTAL FAT (g)
separable lean, cooked	100.00	g	196	32.0	0.0	89.00	338.00	250.00	6.58
	85.05	g	167	27.1	0.0	75.69	287.47	212.62	5.60
	3.00	oz							
liver, pan fried	100.00	g	193	27.4	4.5	85.00	353.00	482.99	6.51
	85.05	g	164	23.3	3.8	72.29	300.22	410.79	5.54
	3.00	oz							
sausage, bratwurst, veal, cooked	100.00	g	341	14.0	0.0	60.00	231.00	150.00	31.70
	83.92	g	286	11.7	0.0	50.35	193.85	125.87	26.60
	2.96	oz							
ground, pan fried	100.00	g	503	8.9	0.9	89.00	107.00	133.00	51.60
	85.05	g	428	7.5	0.8	75.69	91.00	113.12	43.89
	3.00	oz							

VEAL

	SERVING QUANTITY	SERVING UNIT	CALORIES (kCal)	PROTEIN (g)	TOTAL CARBOHYDRATES (g)	SODIUM (mg)	POTASSIUM (mg)	PHOSPHORUS (mg)	TOTAL FAT (g)
sirloin, separable, lean, braised	100.00	g	204	34.0	0.0	81.00	339.00	259.00	6.51
	85.05	g	174	28.9	0.0	68.89	288.32	220.28	5.54
	3.00	oz							
sirloin separable lean, roasted	100.00	g	168	26.3	0.0	85.00	365.00	231.00	6.22
	85.05	g	143	22.4	0.0	72.29	310.43	196.46	5.29
	3.00	oz							
sirloin, lean, raw	100.00	g	110	20.2	0.0	80.00	348.00	220.00	2.59
	113.40	g	125	22.9	0.0	90.72	394.63	249.48	2.94
	4.00	oz							
loin, lean and fat, braised	100.00	g	284	30.2	0.0	80.00	280.00	220.00	17.21
	85.05	g	242	25.7	0.0	68.04	238.14	187.11	14.64
	3.00	oz							
loin, lean and fat, roasted	100.00	g	217	25.0	0.0	93.00	325.00	212.00	12.32
	85.05	g	185	21.1	0.0	79.10	276.41	180.30	10.48
	3.00	oz							
loin, lean, braised	100.00	g	226	33.6	0.0	84.00	297.00	237.00	9.15
	85.05	g	192	28.6	0.0	71.44	252.60	201.57	7.78
	3.00	oz							
loin, lean, roasted	100.00	g	175	26.3	0.0	96.00	340.00	222.00	6.94
	85.05	g	149	22.4	0.0	81.65	289.17	188.81	5.90
	3.00	oz							
loin, lean, raw	100.00	g	114	21.9	0.0	99.00	260.00	237.00	2.90
	113.40	g	129	24.8	0.0	112.27	294.84	268.76	3.29
	4.00	oz							
loin, chop, lean and fat, grilled	100.00	g	198	28.0	0.2	86.00	229.00	208.00	9.48
	85.05	g	168	23.9	0.1	73.14	194.76	176.90	8.06
	3.00	oz							
bratwwurst, veal, cooked	100.00	g	341	14.0	0.0	60.00	231.00	150.00	31.70
	83.92	g	286	11.7	0.0	50.35	193.85	125.87	26.60
	2.96	oz							

SALMON

	SERVING QUANTITY	SERVING UNIT	CALORIES (kcal)	PROTEIN (g)	TOTAL CARBOHYDRATES (g)	SODIUM (mg)	POTASSIUM (mg)	PHOSPHORUS (mg)	TOTAL FAT (g)
pink, raw	100.00	g	127	20.5	0.0	74.99	365.96	260.98	4.40
	113.40	g	144	23.2	0.0	85.04	415.00	295.95	4.99
	4.00	oz							
atlantic, wild, raw	100.00	g	142	19.8	0.0	44.00	489.95	199.98	0.98
	113.40	g	161	22.5	0.0	49.89	555.61	226.78	1.11
	4.00	oz							
atlantic, farmed,raw	100.00	g	208	20.4	0.0	58.99	362.97	239.98	13.42
	113.39	g	236	23.2	0.0	66.90	411.60	272.13	15.22
	4.00	oz							
pink, canned, drained solids, w/ bone	100.00	g	138	23.1	0.0	380.78	332.80	378.78	5.02
	85.05	g	117	19.6	0.0	323.85	283.05	322.15	4.27
	3.00	oz							
pink, canned, with bone and liquid no salt	100.00	g	139	19.8	0.0	75.00	325.99	328.99	6.05
	56.70	g	79	11.2	0.0	42.52	184.84	186.54	3.43
	2.00	oz							
pink, canned, drained solids without skin and bones	100.00	g	136	24.6	0.0	378.00	326.00	253.00	4.21
	85.05	g	116	20.9	0.0	321.49	277.26	215.18	3.58
	3.00	oz							
chum, canned, drained, with bone no salt	100.00	g	141	21.4	0.0	75.00	300.00	353.99	5.50
	56.70	g	80	12.2	0.0	42.52	170.10	200.71	3.12
	2.00	oz							
nuggets, breaded, frozen, heated	100.00	g	212	12.7	14	173.00	165.00	176.00	11.72

TUNA

	SERVING QUANTITY	SERVING UNIT	CALORIES (kcal)	PROTEIN (g)	TOTAL CARBOHYDRATES (g)	SODIUM (mg)	POTASSIUM (mg)	PHOSPHORUS (mg)	TOTAL FAT (g)
bluefin, raw	100.00	g	144	23.3	0.0	39.00	251.98	253.98	4.90
	113.40	g	163	26.5	0.0	44.22	285.74	288.01	5.56
	4.00	oz							
yellowfin or Ahi, raw	100.00	g	109	24.4	0.0	45.00	440.96	277.97	0.49
	113.40	g	124	27.7	0.0	51.03	500.05	315.22	0.56
	4.00	oz							
canned in oil, drained, light no salt	100.00	g	198	29.1	0.0	50.00	207.00	311.00	8.21
	56.70	g	112	16.5	0.0	28.35	117.37	176.33	4.65
	2.00	oz							
white, canned in water, drained no salt	100.00	g	128	23.6	0.0	50.00	237.00	217.00	2.97
	56.70	g	73	13.4	0.0	28.35	134.38	123.04	1.68
	2.00	oz							
canned in water, drained, light no salt	100.00	g	116	25.5	0.0	50.00	237.00	163.00	0.82
	56.70	g	66	14.5	0.0	28.35	134.38	92.42	0.46
	2.00	oz							
white, canned in oil, drained, no salt	100.00	g	186	26.5	0.0	50.00	332.99	267.00	8.08
	56.70	g	105	15.0	0.0	28.35	188.81	151.39	4.58
	2.00	oz							

74

SARDINES	SERVING QUANTITY	SERVING UNIT	CALORIES (kcal)	PROTEIN (g)	TOTAL CARBOHYDRATES (g)	SODIUM (mg)	POTASSIUM (mg)	PHOSPHORUS (mg)	TOTAL FAT (g)
spanish	100.00	g	212	6.2	14.2	310.00	0.00	na	14.16
	113.00	g	240	7.0	16.0	350.00	0.00	na	16.00
	4.00	oz							
atlantic, canned in oil, with bones	100.00	g	208	24.6	0.0	307.00	397.0	490.0	11.45
	24.00	g	50	5.9	0.0	73.68	95.28	117.6	2.75
	2.00	oz							
portuguese	100.00	g	236	25.5	0.0	500.00	na	na	12.73
	55.00	g	130	14.0	0.0	275.00	na	na	7.00
	0.50	c							
fillets, canned	100.00	g	338	18.2	7.3	364.00	na	na	26.36
	55.00	g	186	10.0	4.0	200.00	na	na	14.50
	0.25	c							
TILAPIA									
raw	100.00	g	96	20.1	0.0	52.00	302.0	170.0	1.70
	113.40	g	107	22.8	0.0	58.97	342.5	192.8	1.93
	4.00	oz							
cooked, dry heat	100.00	g	128	26.2	0.0	55.97	379.8	203.9	2.65
	85.05	g	109	22.2	0.0	47.60	323.0	173.4	2.25
	3.00	oz							
POLLOCK									
atlantic, raw	100.00	g	92	19.4	0.0	85.99	355.9	220.9	0.98
	113.40	g	104	22.0	0.0	97.51	403.7	250.6	1.11
	4.00	oz							
atlantic, cooked, dry heat	100.00	g	118	24.9	0.0	110.00	456.0	283.0	1.26
	85.05	g	100	21.2	0.0	93.55	387.8	240.7	1.07
	3.00	oz							
alaska, untreated, cooked	100.00	g	87	19.4	0.0	166.00	364.0	206.0	1.00
	85.05	g	74	16.5	0.0	141.18	309.6	175.2	0.85
	3.00	oz							
PANGASIUS (CREAM DORY/SWAI)									
fillets, boneless	100.00	g	71	14.2	0.0	186.00	na	na	1.77
	113.00	g	80	16.0	0.0	210.00	na	na	2.00
	4.00	oz							
fillets, skinless, boneless	100.00	g	177	20.4	0.0	52.00	na	na	1.77
	113.00	g	200	23.0	0.0	58.80	na	na	2.00
	4.00	oz							

	SERVING QUANTITY	SERVING UNIT	CALORIES (kcal)	PROTEIN (g)	TOTAL CARBOHYDRATES (g)	SODIUM (mg)	POTASSIUM (mg)	PHOSPHORUS (mg)	TOTAL FAT (g)
MUSSELS									
blue, raw	100.00	g	86	11.9	3.7	286.00	320.00	197.00	2.24
	113.40	g	98	13.5	4.2	324.32	362.88	223.40	2.54
	4.00	oz							
blue, cooked,	100.00	g	172	23.8	7.4	369.00	268.00	285.00	4.48
moist heat	85.05	g	146	20.2	6.3	313.83	227.93	242.39	3.81
	3.00	oz							
atlantic or	100.00	g	197	8.8	11.6	415.25	243.87	159.06	12.56
pacific, meat only	85.05	g	167	7.5	9.9	353.17	207.41	1,315	10.69
	3.00	oz							
MACKEREL									
Atlantic or	100.00	g	205	18.6	0.0	89.99	313.97	216.98	13.89
Boston, raw fillet	113.40	g	232	21.1	0.0	102.05	356.04	246.05	15.75
	4.00	oz							
pacific and Jack,	100.00	g	158	20.1	0.0	85.99	405.96	124.99	7.89
raw fillet	113.40	g	179	22.8	0.0	97.51	460.36	141.71	8.95
	4.00	oz							
Atlantic	100.00	g	139	19.3	0.0	58.99	445.96	204.98	6.30
Spanish, raw fillet	113.40	g	158	21.9	0.0	66.90	505.71	232.45	7.14
	4.00	oz							
Jack, canned,	100.00	g	156	23.2	0.0	378.99	194.00	301.00	6.30
solids, drained	56.70	g	88	13.2	0.0	214.89	110.00	170.66	3.57
	2.00	oz							
Atlantic or	100.00	g	262	23.9	0.0	83.00	401.00	278.00	17.81
Boston, cooked, dry heat	85.05	g	223	20.3	0.0	70.59	341.05	236.44	15.15
	3.00	oz							
Atlantic, Spanish, cooked, dry heat	100.00	g	158	23.6	0.0	66.00	553.99	271.00	6.32
	85.05	g	134	20.1	0.0	56.13	471.17	230.48	5.38
	3.00	oz							
Pacific and Jack,	100.00	g	201	25.7	0.0	110.00	520.99	160.00	10.12
mixed species, cooked	85.05	g	171	21.9	0.0	93.55	443.11	136.08	8.61
	3.00	oz							

	SERVING QUANTITY	SERVING UNIT	CALORIES (kcal)	PROTEIN (g)	TOTAL CARBOHYDRATES (g)	SODIUM (mg)	POTASSIUM (mg)	PHOSPHORUS (mg)	TOTAL FAT (g)
TROUT									
rainbow, wild, *raw, fillet*	100.00	g	119	20.5	0.0	31.00	481.00	271.00	3.46
	113.40	g	135	23.2	0.0	35.15	545.45	307.31	3.92
	4.00	oz							
rainbow, farmed, *raw, fillet*	100.00	g	141	19.9	0.0	51.00	376.96	225.98	6.18
	113.40	g	160	22.6	0.0	57.83	427.48	256.26	7.01
	4.00	oz							
mixed species, raw fillet	100.00	g	148	20.8	0.0	52.00	360.97	244.98	6.61
	113.40	g	168	23.6	0.0	58.96	409.33	277.80	7.50
	4.00	oz							
sea trout, *mixed species, raw*	100.00	g	104	16.7	0.0	57.99	340.97	249.98	3.61
	113.40	g	118	19.0	0.0	65.77	386.66	283.47	4.09
	4.00	oz							
rainbow, wild, *cooked, dry heat*	100.00	g	150	22.9	0.0	56.00	448.00	269.00	5.82
	85.05	g	128	19.5	0.0	47.63	381.02	228.78	4.95
	3.00	oz							
rainbow, farmed, *cooked, dry heat*	100.00	g	168	23.8	0.0	61.00	450.00	270.00	7.38
	85.05	g	143	20.2	0.0	51.88	382.72	229.63	6.28
	3.00	oz							
mixed species, *cooked, dry heat*	100.00	g	190	26.6	0.0	67.00	463.00	314.00	8.47
	85.05	g	162	22.7	0.0	56.98	393.78	267.05	7.20
	3.00	oz							
sea trout, mixed species, *cooked, dry heat*	100.00	g	133	21.5	0.0	74.00	437.00	321.00	4.63
	85.05	g	113	18.3	0.0	62.94	371.66	273.01	3.94
	3.00	oz							
CARP									
raw	100.00	g	127	17.8	0.0	49.00	332.97	414.96	5.60
	113.40	g	144	20.2	0.0	55.56	377.59	470.56	6.35
	4.00	oz							
cooked, dry heat	100.00	g	162	22.9	0.0	63.00	427.00	530.99	7.17
	85.05	g	138	19.4	0.0	53.58	363.16	451.61	6.10
	3.00	oz							
MAHI-MAHI									
Dorado or Dolphinfish, raw	100.00	g	85	18.5	0.0	87.99	415.96	142.99	0.70
	113.40	g	96	21.0	0.0	99.78	471.70	162.15	0.79
	4.00	oz							
Doradao or Dolphinfish, *cooked, dry heat*	100.00	g	109	23.7	0.0	113.00	532.99	183.00	0.90
	85.05	g	93	20.2	0.0	96.11	452.31	155.64	0.77
	3.00	oz							

FLATFISH	SERVING QUANTITY	SERVING UNIT	CALORIES (kcal)	PROTEIN (g)	TOTAL CARBOHYDRATES (g)	SODIUM (mg)	POTASSIUM (mg)	PHOSPHORUS (mg)	TOTAL FAT (g)
raw	100.00	g	70	12.4	0.0	295.97	159.98	251.98	1.93
	113.40	g	79	14.1	0.0	335.63	181.42	285.74	2.19
	4.00	oz							
cooked, dry	100.00	g	86	15.2	0.0	363.00	197.00	309.00	2.37
heat	85.05	g	73	13.0	0.0	308.73	167.55	262.80	2.02
	3.00	oz							
HALIBUT									
greenland, raw	100.00	g	186	14.4	0.0	79.99	267.97	163.98	13.84
	113.40	g	211	16.3	0.0	90.71	303.88	185.96	15.69
	4.00	oz							
atlantic and	100.00	g	91	18.6	0.0	67.99	434.96	235.98	1.33
pacific, raw	113.40	g	103	21.0	0.0	77.10	493.24	267.60	1.51
	4.00	oz							
greenland,	100.00	g	239	18.4	0.0	103.00	344.00	210.00	17.71
cooked, dry heat	85.05	g	203	15.7	0.0	87.60	292.57	178.60	15.09
	3.00	oz							
atlantic and	100.00	g	111	22.5	0.0	82.00	527.99	287.00	1.61
pacific, cooked, dry heat	85.05	g	94	19.2	0.0	69.74	449.06	244.09	1.37
	3.00	oz							
LOBSTER									
Northern, raw	100.00	g	77	16.5	0.0	423.00	200.00	161.00	0.75
(Langoustine)	113.40	g	87	18.7	0.0	479.68	226.80	182.57	0.85
	4.00	Oz							
Spiny, mixed	100.00	g	112	20.6	2.4	177.00	180.00	238.00	1.51
species, raw	113.40	g	127	23.4	2.8	200.72	104.12	269.89	1.71
	4.00	oz							
Northern, cooked, moist	100.00	g	89	19.0	0.0	485.99	230.00	185.00	0.86
heat	85.05	g	76	16.2	0.0	413.34	195.61	157.34	0.73
(Langoustine)									
	3.00	oz							
Spiny, mixed	100.00	g	143	26.4	3.1	227.00	208.00	229.00	1.94
species, cooked, moist heat	85.05	g	122	22.5	2.7	193.06	176.90	194.76	1.65
	3.00	oz							

	SERVING QUANTITY	SERVING UNIT	CALORIES (kCal)	PROTEIN (g)	TOTAL CARBOHYDRATES (g)	SODIUM (mg)	POTASSIUM (mg)	PHOSPHORUS (mg)	TOTAL FAT (g)
COD									
atlantic, raw	100.00	g	82	17.8	0.0	54.00	412.96	202.98	0.67
	113.40	g	93	20.2	0.0	61.23	468.30	230.18	0.76
	4.00	oz							
atlantic, canned	100.00	g	105	22.8	0.0	218.00	527.99	260.00	0.86
	56.70	g	60	12.9	0.0	123.60	299.37	147.42	0.49
	2.00	oz							
atlantic,	100.00	g	105	22.8	0.0	78.00	244.00	138.00	0.86
cooked, dry heat	85.05	g	89	19.4	0.0	66.34	207.52	117.37	0.73
	3.00	oz							
pacific, raw	100.00	g	69	15.3	0.0	302.97	234.98	280.97	0.41
	113.40	g	78	17.3	0.0	343.57	266.46	318.62	0.46
	4.00	oz							
pacific, cooked,	100.00	g	85	18.7	0.0	372.00	289.00	345.00	0.50
dry heat	85.05	g	72	15.9	0.0	316.38	245.79	293.42	0.43
	3.00	oz							
ANCHOVIES									
Raw	100.00	g	131	20.4	0.0	103.99	382.96	173.98	4.84
	113.40	g	149	23.1	0.0	117.92	434.28	197.30	5.49
	4.00	oz							
canned, in oil,	100.00	g	210	28.9	0.0	3,668	544.00	252.00	9.71
drained	16.00	g	34	4.6	0.0	586.88	87.04	40.32	1.55
	4.00	pcs							
SHRIMP									
mixed species,	100.00	g	71	13.6	0.9	566.00	113.00	244.00	1.01
raw	113.40	g	81	15.4	1.0	641.84	128.14	276.40	1.15
	4.00	oz							
mixed species,	100.00	g	242	21.4	12	343.80	224.87	217.87	12.27
breaded, fried	85.05	g	206	18.2	9.8	292.40	191.25	185.30	10.44
	3.00	oz							
mixed species,	100.00	g	119	22.8	1.5	946.99	170.00	306.00	1.70
cooked, moist heat	85.05	g	101	19.4	1.3	805.41	144.58	260.25	1.45
	3.00	oz							
cracker	100.00	g	426	7.1	59	571.00	193.00	191.00	17.86

CRAB

	SERVING QUANTITY	SERVING UNIT	CALORIES (kcal)	PROTEIN (g)	TOTAL CARBOHYDRATES (g)	SODIUM (mg)	POTASSIUM (mg)	PHOSPHORUS (mg)	TOTAL FAT (g)
blue, raw	100.0	g	87	18.1	0.0	293.00	329.00	229.00	1.08
	113.4	g	99	20.5	0.5	332.26	373.09	259.69	1.22
	4.00	oz							
blue, canned	100.0	g	83	17.9	0.0	562.99	259.00	234.00	0.74
	56.70	g	47	10.1	0.0	319.22	146.85	132.68	0.42
	2.00	oz							
dungeness, raw	100.0	g	86	17.4	0.7	295.00	354.00	182.00	0.97
	113.4	g	98	19.7	0.8	334.53	401.44	206.39	1.10
	4.00	oz							
dungeness, cooked, moist heat	100.0	g	110	22.3	1.0	378.00	408.00	175.00	1.24
	85.05	g	94	19.0	0.8	321.49	347.00	148.84	1.05
	3.00	oz							
alaska king, raw	100.0	g	84	18.3	0.0	836.00	204.00	219.00	0.60
	113.4	g	95	20.7	0.0	948.02	231.34	248.35	0.68
	4.00	oz							
alaska king, cooked, moist heat	100.0	g	97	19.4	0.0	1,072	262.00	280.00	1.54
	85.05	g	83	16.5	0.0	911.73	222.83	238.14	1.31
	3.00	oz							
imitation, crabmeat (Kani)	100.0	g	95	7.6	15.0	528.99	90.00	282.00	0.46
	85.05	g	81	6.5	12.8	449.91	76.54	239.84	0.39
	3.00	Oz							
cakes	100.0	g	266	18.8	8.5	819.00	270.00	378.00	17.25
	60.00	g	160	11.3	5.1	491.00	162.00	226.80	10.35
	1.00	pc							

CATFISH

	SERVING QUANTITY	SERVING UNIT	CALORIES (kcal)	PROTEIN (g)	TOTAL CARBOHYDRATES (g)	SODIUM (mg)	POTASSIUM (mg)	PHOSPHORUS (mg)	TOTAL FAT (g)
channel, wild, raw	100.0	g	95	16.4	0.0	43.00	405.93	208.98	2.82
	113.4	g	108	18.6	0.0	48.76	357.97	236.98	3.20
	4.00	oz							
channel, farmed, raw	100.0	g	119	15.2	0.0	97.94	301.82	203.88	5.94
	85.05	g	101	13.0	0.0	83.30	256.70	173.40	5.05
	3.00	oz							
breaded, fried	100.0	g	229	18.1	8.0	280.00	340.00	216.00	13.33
	85.05	g	195	15.4	6.8	238.14	289.17	183.71	11.34
	3.00	oz							
wild, cooked, dry heat	100.0	g	105	18.5	0.0	50.00	419.00	304.00	2.85
	85.05	g	89	15.7	0.0	42.52	356.36	258.55	2.42
	3.00	oz							
farmed, cooked, dry heat	100.0	g	144	18.4	0.0	119.00	366.00	247.00	7.19
	85.05	g	122	15.7	0.0	101.21	311.28	210.07	6.12
	3.00	oz							

CRAYFISH/ CRAWFISH	SERVING QUANTITY	SERVING UNIT	CALORIES (kcal)	PROTEIN (g)	TOTAL CARBOHYDRATES (g)	SODIUM (mg)	POTASSIUM (mg)	PHOSPHORUS (mg)	TOTAL FAT (g)
Mixed species, farmed, raw	100.00	g	72	14.9	0.0	62.00	261.00	218.00	0.97
	113.40 4.00	g oz	82	16.8	0.0	70.31	295.97	247.21	1.10
Mixed species, wild, raw	100.00	g	77	16.0	0.0	58.00	302.00	256.00	0.95
	113.40 4.00	g oz	87	18.1	0.0	65.77	342.47	290.30	1.08
Mixed species, farmed, cooked, moist heat	100.00	g	87	17.5	0.0	97.00	238.00	241.00	0.22
	85.05 3.00	g oz	74	14.9	0.0	82.50	202.42	204.97	0.18
mixed species, wild, cooked, moist heat	100.00	g	82	16.8	0.0	94.00	296.00	270.00	1.20
	85.05 3.00	g oz	70	14.3	0.0	79.95	251.75	229.63	1.02

SQUID (CALAMARI)

mixed species, fried	100.00	g	175	17.9	7.8	306.0	279.00	251.00	7.48
	85.05 3.00	g oz	149	15.3	6.6	260.3	237.29	213.47	6.36
mixed species, raw	100.00	g	92	15.6	3.1	44.00	246.00	221.00	1.38
boneless	113.40 4.00	g oz	104	17.7	3.5	49.90	278.96	250.61	1.56

81

CLAMS

	SERVING QUANTITY	SERVING UNIT	CALORIES (kcal)	PROTEIN (g)	TOTAL CARBOHYDRATES (g)	SODIUM (mg)	POTASSIUM (mg)	PHOSPHORUS (mg)	TOTAL FAT (g)
mixed species, raw	100	g	86	14.7	3.6	601.00	46.00	198.00	0.96
	85.05	g	73	12.5	3.0	511.15	39.12	168.40	0.82
	3.00	oz							
mixed species, breaded, fried	100.00	g	202	14.2	10.3	364.00	326.00	188.00	11.15
	85.05	g	172	12.1	8.8	309.58	277.26	159.89	9.48
	3.00	oz							
mixed species, canned, with liquid	100.00	g	2	0.4	0.1	215.00	149.00	114.00	0.02
	28.35	g	1	0.1	0.0	60.95	42.24	32.32	0.01
	1.00	oz							
mixed species, canned, drained	100.00	g	142	24.3	5.9	112.00	627.99	326.99	1.59
	56.70	g	81	13.8	3.4	63.50	356.07	185.41	0.90
	2.00	oz							

OYSTERS

	SERVING QUANTITY	SERVING UNIT	CALORIES (kcal)	PROTEIN (g)	TOTAL CARBOHYDRATES (g)	SODIUM (mg)	POTASSIUM (mg)	PHOSPHORUS (mg)	TOTAL FAT (g)
ostrich, raw	100.00	g	125	21.6	0.0	83.00	297.00	204.00	3.67
	85.05	g	106	18.3	0.0	70.59	252.60	173.50	3.12
	3.00	oz							
ostrich, cooked	100.00	g	159	28.8	0.0	81.00	409.00	281.00	3.97
	85.05	g	135	24.5	0.0	68.89	347.85	238.99	3.38
	3.00	oz							
pacific, raw	100.00	g	81	9.5	5.0	106.00	168.00	162.00	2.30
	113.40	g	92	10.7	5.6	120.20	190.51	183.71	2.61
	4.00	oz							
pacific, cooked, moist heat	100.00	g	163	18.9	9.9	212.00	302.00	243.00	4.60
	85.05	g	139	16.1	8.4	180.30	256.85	206.67	3.91
	3.00	oz							
eastern, canned	100.00	g	68	7.1	3.9	112.00	229.00	139.00	2.47
	56.70	g	39	4.0	2.2	63.50	129.84	78.81	1.40
	2.00	oz							
eastern, farmed, raw	100.00	g	59	5.2	5.5	178.00	124.00	93.00	1.55
	85.05	g	50	4.4	4.7	151.39	105.46	79.10	1.32
	3.00	oz							
eastern, wild, raw	100.00	g	51	5.7	2.7	85.00	156.00	97.00	1.71
	113.40	g	58	6.5	3.1	96.39	176.90	110.00	1.94
	4.00	oz							
eastern, wild, breaded, fried	100.00	g	199	8.8	11.6	417.00	244.00	159.00	12.58
	85.05	g	169	7.5	9.9	354.65	207.52	135.23	10.70
	3.00	oz							
battered, breaded, fried, fast food	100.00	g	265	9.0	28.7	486.99	131.00	141.00	12.90
	85.05	g	225	7.7	24.4	414.19	111.41	119.92	10.97
	3.00	oz							

	SERVING QUANTITY	SERVING UNIT	CALORIES (kcal)	PROTEIN (g)	TOTAL CARBOHYDRATES (g)	SODIUM (mg)	POTASSIUM (mg)	PHOSPHORUS (mg)	TOTAL FAT (g)
SCALLOPS									
Mixed species, raw	100.00	g	69	12.1	3.2	392.00	205.00	12.80	0.49
	113.40	g	78	13.7	3.6	444.53	232.47	14.52	0.56
	4.00	oz							
Bay and Sea, steamed	100.00	g	111	20.5	5.4	667.00	314.00	426.00	0.84
	85.05	g	94	17.5	4.6	567.28	267.06	362.31	0.71
	3.00	oz							
mixed species, breaded and fried	100.00	g	216	18.1	10.1	464.00	333.00	236.00	10.94
	46.50	g	100	8.4	4.7	215.76	15.85	109.74	5.09
	3.00	pcs							
breaded, fried, fast food	100.00	g	268	10.9	26.7	637.99	204.00	203.00	13.47
	85.05	g	228	9.3	22.7	542.61	173.50	172.65	11.46
	3.00	oz							
HERRING									
Pacific, raw	100.00	g	195	16.4	0.0	73.99	422.96	227.98	13.88
	113.40	g	221	18.6	0.0	83.91	479.64	258.53	15.74
	4.00	oz							
Atlantic, raw	100.00	g	158	18.0	0.0	89.99	326.97	235.98	9.04
	113.40	g	179	20.4	0.0	102.05	370.78	267.60	10.25
	4.00	oz							
Pacific, cooked, dry heat	100.00	g	250	21.0	0.0	95.00	541.99	292.00	17.79
	85.05	g	213	17.9	0.0	80.80	460.97	248.34	15.13
	3.00	oz							
Atlantic, cooked, dry heat	100.00	g	203	23.0	0.0	115.00	419.00	303.00	11.49
	85.05	g	173	19.6	0.0	97.81	356.36	257.70	9.86
	3.00	oz							
Roe or eggs, Pacific (Alaska Native)	100.00	g	74	9.6	4.5	61.00	na	na	1.93
	85.05	g	63	8.2	3.8	51.88	na	na	1.64
	3.00	oz							

C. Milk and Cheeses

(Dairy and Non-Dairy)

Hey there!

Do you need to print out this Food List?

You can download a printable version of this chart by scanning the QR code below or copying the link on your computer browser.

https://go.renaltracker.com/printfoodlist

MILK

MILK	SERVING QUANTITY	SERVING UNIT	CALORIES (Kcal)	PROTEIN (g)	TOTAL CARBOHYDRATES (g)	SODIUM (mg)	POTASSIUM (mg)	PHOSPHORUS (mg)	TOTAL FAT (g)
(cow) whole	100	g	60	3.3	4.7	38.0	150.0	101.0	3.20
	244	g	146	8.0	11.4	92.7	366.0	246.0	7.81
	1	c							
2% reduced fat	100	g	50	3.4	4.9	39.0	159.0	103.0	1.90
	244	g	122	8.2	12.0	95.2	388.0	251.0	4.64
	1	c							
low fat (1%)	100	g	43	3.4	5.2	39.0	159.0	103.0	0.95
	244	g	105	8.3	12.7	95.2	388.0	251.0	2.32
	1	c							
skim, fat free	100	g	34	3.4	4.9	41.0	167.0	107.0	0.08
	244	g	83	8.4	11.9	100.0	407.0	261.0	0.20
	1	c							
lactose free, from whole milk	100	g	60	3.3	4.7	38.0	150.0	101.0	3.20
	244	g	146	8.0	11.4	92.7	366.0	246.0	7.81
	1	c							
Buttermilk, dried	100	g	387	34.3	49.0	517.0	1592	933	5.78
	6.5	g	25	2.2	3.2	33.6	103.0	60.60	0.38
	1	tbsp							
buttermilk, fluid, whole	100	g	62	3.2	4.9	105.0	135.0	85.00	3.31
	245	g	152	7.9	12.0	257.0	331.0	208.0	8.11
	1	c							
condensed, sweetened	100	g	321	7.9	54.4	127.0	371.0	253.0	8.70
	38	g	122	3.0	20.7	48.3	141.0	96.10	3.31
	1	fl oz							
evaporated, whole	100	g	134	6.8	10.0	106.0	303.0	203.0	7.56
	31.5	g	42	2.1	3.2	33.4	95.40	63.90	2.38
	1	fl oz							
malted	100	g	64	3.2	8.7	60.0	150.0	98.00	1.91
	256	g	164	8.2	22.2	154.0	384.0	251.0	4.89
	1	c							
chocolate	100	g	67	3.4	13.5	79.0	182.0	101.0	0.00
	248	g	166	8.4	33.4	196.0	451.0	250.0	0.00
	1	c							
strawberry (whole milk)	100	g	85	3.0	11.8	38.0	139.0	94.00	2.97
	248	g	211	7.5	29.3	94.2	345.0	233.0	7.37
	1	c							

MILK

	SERVING QUANTITY	SERVING UNIT	CALORIES (kcal)	PROTEIN (g)	TOTAL CARBOHYDRATES (g)	SODIUM (mg)	POTASSIUM (mg)	PHOSPHORUS (mg)	TOTAL FAT (g)
SOY	100	g	43	2.6	4.9	47.0	122.0	43.00	1.47
	244	g	105	6.3	12.0	115.0	298.0	105.0	3.59
	1	c							
soy, light	100	g	30	2.4	3.5	48.0	117.0	87.00	0.77
	244	g	73	5.8	8.6	117.0	285.0	212.0	1.88
	1	c							
soy, chocolate	100	g	63	2.3	10.0	53.0	143.0	51.00	1.53
	244	g	154	5.5	24.3	129.0	349.0	124.0	3.73
	1	c							
soy, non-fat	100	g	28	2.5	4.1	57.0	105.0	87.00	0.04
	244	g	68	6.0	10.1	139.0	256.0	212.0	0.10
	1	c							
RICE	100	g	47	0.3	9.2	39.0	27.00	56.00	0.97
	244	g	115	0.7	22.4	95.2	65.90	137.0	2.37
	1	c							
rice milk, unsweetened	100	g	47	0.3	9.2	39.0	27.00	56.00	0.97
	240	g	113	0.7	22.0	93.6	64.80	134.0	2.33
	8	fl oz							
ALMOND, unsweeteened	100	g	15	0.4	1.3	72.0	67.00	9.00	0.96
	244	g	37	1.0	3.2	176.0	163.0	22.00	2.34
	1	c							
almond, unsweetened, chocolate	100	g	16	0.5	1.5	72.0	71.00	11.00	1.00
	244	g	39	1.1	3.6	176.0	173.0	26.80	2.44
	1	c							
almond milk, sweeteend	100	g	30	0.4	5.2	69.0	64.00	9.00	0.93
	244	g	73	0.9	12.8	168.0	156.0	22.00	2.27
	1	c							
almond, sweetened, chocolate	100	g	41	0.4	8.3	67.0	67.00	11.00	0.95
	244	g	100	1.1	20.4	163.0	163.0	26.80	2.32
	1	c							
COCONUT	100	g	31	0.2	2.9	19.0	19.00	0.00	2.08
	244	g	76	0.5	7.1	46.4	46.40	0.00	5.08
	1	c							
GOAT, whole	100	g	69	3.6	4.5	50.0	204.0	111.0	4.14
	244	g	168	8.7	10.9	122.0	498.0	271.0	10.10
	1	c							

MILK SUBSTITUTE	SERVING QUANTITY	SERVING UNIT	CALORIES (KCal)	PROTEIN (g)	TOTAL CARBOHYDRATES (g)	SODIUM (mg)	POTASSIUM (mg)	PHOSPHORUS (mg)	TOTAL FAT (g)
Non-dairy milk/creamer	100	g	29	1.0	3.8	60.0	80.00	19.00	1.17
	30.5 1	g fl oz	9	0.3	1.1	18.3	24.40	5.80	0.36
imitation, non-soy	100	g	46	1.6	5.3	55.0	150.0	100.0	2.00
	244 1	g cup	112	3.9	12.9	134.0	366.0	244.0	4.88
Kefir	100	g	52	3.6	7.5	38.0	159.0	100.0	0.96
	244 1	g c	127	8.8	18.3	92.7	388.0	244	2.34
Sorbet	100	g	110	0.8	27.1	13.0	28.00	3.00	0.05
	80 1	g bar	88	0.6	21.7	10.4	22.40	2.40	0.04

YOGURT	SERVING QUANTITY	SERVING UNIT	CALORIES (KCal)	PROTEIN (g)	TOTAL CARBOHYDRATES (g)	SODIUM (mg)	POTASSIUM (mg)	PHOSPHORUS (mg)	TOTAL FAT (g)
coconut milk, yogurt	100	g	64	0.3	8.0	21.0	27.00	2.00	3.50
	170 6	g oz	109	0.5	13.5	35.7	45.90	3.40	5.95
dressing	100	g	220	3.5	11.8	43.0	146.0	85.00	18.27
	15.4 1	g tbsp	34	0.5	1.8	6.6	22.50	13.10	2.81
liquid	100	g	72	3.7	11.8	53.0	171.0	103.0	1.09
	245 1	g c	176	9.1	28.9	130.0	419.0	252.0	2.67
plain, whole milk	100	g	61	3.5	4.7	46.0	155.0	95.00	3.25
	227 8	g oz	138	7.9	10.6	104.0	352.0	216.0	7.38
Whole milk with fruit	100	g	87 14	3.1	12.4	44.0	146.0	86.00	2.87
	170 6	g oz	8	5.3	21.0	74.8	248.0	146.0	4.88

YOGURT

YOGURT	SERVING QUANTITY	SERVING UNIT	CALORIES (kcal)	PROTEIN (g)	TOTAL CARBOHYDRATES (g)	SODIUM (mg)	POTASSIUM (mg)	PHOSPHORUS (mg)	TOTAL FAT (g)
whole milk, flavored (non-fruit)	100	g	77	3.3	9.4	44.0	147.0	90.00	3.10
	170	g	131	5.6	16.0	74.8	250.0	153.0	5.27
	6	oz							
non-fat milk, plain, vanilla	100	g	78	2.9	17.0	47.0	141.0	88.00	0.00
	227	g	177	6.7	38.7	107.0	320.0	200.0	0.00
	8	oz							
non-fat milk, fruit	100	g	83	5.1	15.0	72.0	234.0	140.0	0.17
	170	g	141	8.7	25.5	122.0	398.0	238.0	0.29
	6	oz							
Soy, yogurt, plain	100	g	94	3.5	16.0	35.0	47.00	38.00	1.80
	170	g	160	6.0	27.1	59.5	79.90	64.60	3.06
	6	oz							
Greek, plain, whole milk	100	g	97	9.0	4.0	35.0	141.0	135.0	5.00
	170	g	165	15.3	6.8	59.5	240.0	230.0	8.50
	6	oz							
Greek, fruit, whole milk	100	g	106	7.3	12.3	37.0	113.0	109.0	3.00
	170	g	180	12.5	20.9	62.9	192.0	185.0	5.10
	6	oz							
Greek, flavored, other than fruit	100	g	111	8.5	9.4	39.0	121.0	117.0	4.44
	170	g	189	14.4	15.9	66.3	206.0	199.0	7.55
	6	oz							
Greek, plain, low fat	100	g	73	10.0	3.9	34.0	141.0	137.0	1.92
	170	g	124	16.9	6.7	57.8	240.0	233.0	3.26
	6	oz							
Greek, LF, flavors other than fruit	100	g	95	8.6	9.5	40.0	123.0	119.0	2.50
	170	g	162	14.7	16.2	68.0	209.0	202.0	4.25
	6	oz							
Greek, non-fat (NF), plain	100	g	59	10.2	3.6	36.0	141.0	135.0	0.39
	170	g	100	17.3	6.1	61.2	240.0	230.0	0.66
	6	oz							
Greek, NF, flavors other than fruit	100	g	78	8.6	10.4	34.0	123.0	119.0	0.18
	170	g	133	14.7	17.6	57.8	209.0	202.0	0.31
	6	oz							
Frozen yogurt, chocolate 1 scoop= small cup	100	g	131	3.0	21.6	63.0	234.0	89.00	3.60
	160	g	210	4.8	34.6	101.0	374.0	142.0	5.76
	1	scoop							

YOGURT

	SERVING QUANTITY	SERVING UNIT	CALORIES (kcal)	PROTEIN (g)	TOTAL CARBOHYDRATES (g)	SODIUM (mg)	POTASSIUM (mg)	PHOSPHORUS (mg)	TOTAL FAT (g)
Frozen yogurt, *vanilla*	100	g	127	3.0	21.6	63.0	156.0	89.00	3.60
	160	g	203	4.8	34.6	101.0	250.0	142.0	5.76
1 scoop= small cup	1	scoop							
Frozen yogurt, soft serve, *chocolate*	100	g	160	4.3	24.9	86.0	237.0	141.0	5.76
	175	g	280	7.5	43.5	150.0	415.0	247.0	10.10
	1	c							
Frozn yogurt, soft serve, *vanilla*	100	g	159	4.0	24.2	87.0	211.0	129.0	5.60
	175	g	278	7.0	42.4	152.0	369.0	226.0	9.80
	1	c							
Frozn yogurt bar, *vanilla*	100	g	127	3.0	21.6	63.0	156.0	89.00	3.60
	65	g	83	2.0	14.0	41.0	101.0	57.80	2.34
	1	bar							
Frozn yogurt bar, *chocolate*	100	g	131	3.0	21.6	63.0	234.0	89.00	3.60
	65	g	85	2.0	14.0	41.0	152.0	57.80	2.34
	1	bar							
Frozn yogurt cone, *vanilla*	100	g	139	3.2	23.9	71.0	154.0	89.00	3.73
	125	g	174	4.0	29.9	88.8	192.0	111.0	4.66
	1	cone							
Frozn yogurt cone, *chocolate*	100	g	142	3.2	23.9	71.0	229.0	89.00	3.73
	125	g	178	4.0	29.9	88.8	286.0	111.0	4.66
	1	cone							
Frozn yogurt, *waffle* cone, *vanilla*	100	g	143	3.3	25.3	77.0	155.0	90.00	3.61
	255	g	365	8.4	64.5	196.0	395.0	230.0	9.20
	1	cone							
Frozn yogurt, *waffle* cone, *choco*	100	g	147	3.3	25.3	77.0	229.0	90.00	3.61
	255	g	375	8.4	64.5	196.0	584.0	230.0	9.20
	1	cone							

CHEESE

	SERVING QUANTITY	SERVING UNIT	CALORIES (kcal)	PROTEIN (g)	TOTAL CARBOHYDRATES (g)	SODIUM (mg)	POTASSIUM (mg)	PHOSPHORUS (mg)	TOTAL FAT (g)
mozzarella, from whole milk	100	g	299	22.2	2.4	486.0	76.00	354.0	22.14
shredded	112	g	335	24.8	2.7	544.0	85.10	396.0	24.80
	1	c							
mozzarella, part	100	g	254	24.3	2.8	619.0	84.00	463.0	15.92
skim milk	28.35	g	72	6.9	0.8	175.0	23.80	131.0	4.51
	1	oz							
Mozzarella, reduced sodium	100	g	280	27.5	3.1	16.0	95.00	524.0	17.10
(shredded)	113	g	316	31.1	3.5	18.1	107.0	592.0	19.30
	1	cup							
ricotta, from	100	g	158	7.8	6.9	105.0	230.0	162.0	11.00
whole milk	129	g	204	10.1	8.9	135.0	297.0	209.0	14.20
	0.5	c							
riccota, part	100	g	138	11.4	5.1	99.0	125.0	183.0	7.91
skim milk	124	g	171	14.1	6.4	123.0	155.0	227.0	9.81
	0.5	c							
cream cheese,	100	g	295	7.1	3.5	436.0	112.0	91.00	28.60
regular	28.35	g	84	2.0	1.0	124.0	31.80	25.80	8.11
	1	oz							
cream cheese,	100	g	201	7.9	8.1	359.0	247.0	152.0	15.28
light	28.35	g	57	2.2	2.3	102.0	70.00	43.10	4.33
	1	oz							
processed	100	g	307	16.1	8.9	1279.0	295.0	768.0	23.06
cheese food	21	g	65	3.4	1.9	269.0	62.00	161.0	4.84
	1	slice							
Cottage cheese	100	g	84	11.0	4.3	321.0	120.0	148.0	2.30
	210	g	176	23.1	9.1	674.0	252.0	311.0	4.83
	1	cup							
cottage cheese.	100	g	84	11.0	4.3	321.0	120.0	148.0	2.30
low fat	226	g	190	24.9	9.7	725.0	271.0	334.0	5.20
	1	cup							
Monterey	100	g	373	24.5	0.7	600.0	81.00	444.0	30.28
shredded	113	g	421	27.7	0.8	678.0	91.50	502.0	34.20
	1	cup							
Cheddar	100	g	408	23.3	2.4	654.0	77.00	458.0	34.00
	21	g	86	4.9	0.5	137.0	16.20	96.20	7.14
	1	slice							

CHEESE	SERVING QUANTITY	SERVING UNIT	CALORIES (kcal)	PROTEIN (g)	TOTAL CARBOHYDRATES (g)	SODIUM (mg)	POTASSIUM (mg)	PHOSPHORUS (mg)	TOTAL FAT (g)
Cheddar, reduced sodium	100	g	398	24.4	1.9	21.0	112.00	484.0	32.62
	21	g	84	5.1	0.4	4.4	23.50	102.0	6.85
	1	slice							
Cheddar, sharp sliced	100	g	410	24.3	2.1	644.0	76.00	460.0	33.82
	28	g	115	6.8	0.6	180.0	21.30	129.0	9.47
	1	oz							
Cheddar/ American cheese spread	100	g	290	16.4	8.7	1625	242.00	875.0	21.23
	21	g	61	3.5	1.8	341.0	50.80	184.0	4.46
	1	wedge							
American	100	g	307	16.1	8.9	1279.	295.00	768.0	23.06
	21	g	65	3.4	1.9	269.0	62.00	161.0	4.84
	1	slice							
Brick	100	g	371	23.2	2.8	560.0	136.00	451.0	29.68
	17.2	g	64	4.0	0.5	96.3	23.40	77.60	5.10
	1	cubic inch							
Brie	100	g	334	20.8	0.5	629.0	152.00	188.0	27.68
	17	g	57	3.5	0.1	107.0	25.80	32.00	4.71
	1	cubic inch							
blue	100	g	353	21.4	2.3	1146	256.00	387.0	28.74
	28.35	g	100	6.1	0.7	325.0	72.60	110.0	8.15
	1	oz							
Camembert	100	g	300	19.8	0.5	842.0	187.00	347.0	24.26
	38	g	114	7.5	0.2	320.0	71.10	132.0	9.22
1 wedge = 1.33 oz	1	wedge							
Colby	100	g	394	23.8	2.6	604.0	127.00	457.0	32.11
	21	g	83	5.0	0.5	127.0	26.70	96.00	6.74
	1	slice							
Caraway	100	g	376	25.2	1.1	690.0	93.00	490.0	29.20
	28.35	g	107	7.1	0.9	196.0	26.40	139.0	8.28
	1	oz							
Edam	100	g	356	24.9	2.2	819.0	121.00	546.0	27.44
	21	g	75	5.2	0.5	172.0	25.40	115.0	5.76
	1	slice							
Feta	100	g	265	14.2	3.9	1139.	62.00	337.0	21.49
	17	g	45	2.4	0.7	194.0	10.50	57.30	3.62
	1	cubic inch							
Fontina	100	g	389	25.6	1.6	800.0	64.00	346.0	31.14
	21	g	82	5.4	0.3	168.0	13.40	72.70	6.54
	1	slice							
goat	100	g	364	21.6	0.1	415.0	158.00	375.0	29.84
	25	g	91	5.4	0.0	104.0	39.50	93.80	7.46
	1	cubic inch							

CHEESE

	SERVING QUANTITY	SERVING UNIT	CALORIES (kcal)	PROTEIN (g)	TOTAL CARBOHYDRATES (g)	SODIUM (mg)	POTASSIUM (mg)	PHOSPHORUS (mg)	TOTAL FAT (g)
Gouda	100	g	356	24.9	2.2	819.0	121.0	546.0	27.44
	28.35	g	101	7.0	0.6	232.0	34.30	155.0	7.78
	1	oz							
Gruyere	100	g	413	29.8	0.4	714.0	81.00	605.0	32.34
	21	g	87	6.3	0.1	150.0	17.00	127.0	6.70
	1	slice							
Blue or Roquefort	100	g	353	21.4	2.3	1146.0	256.0	387.0	28.74
	17.3	g	61	3.7	0.4	198.0	44.30	67.00	4.97
	1	cubic inch							
Colby Jack	100	g	384	24.1	1.6	602.0	104.0	450.0	31.20
	21	g	81	5.1	0.3	126.0	21.80	94.50	6.55
	1	slice							
Parmesan, grated	100	g	420	29.6	12.4	1750.0	184.0	634.0	28.00
	7.6	g	32	2.3	0.9	133.0	14.00	48.20	1.82
	1	tbsp							
Parmesan, hard	100	g	421	29.6	12.4	1750.0	184.0	634.0	28.00
	10.3	g	43	3.1	1.3	180.0	19.00	65.30	2.88
	1	cubic inch							
Mexican blend shredded	100	g	358	23.5	1.8	607.0	85.00	438.0	28.51
	113	g	405	26.6	2.0	686.0	96.00	495.0	32.20
	1	cup							
Mexican blend, reduced fat shredded	100	g	282	24.7	3.4	776.0	93.00	583.0	19.40
	113	g	319	27.9	3.9	877.0	105.0	659.0	21.90
	1	cup							
Muenster	100	g	368	23.4	1.1	628.0	134.0	468.0	30.04
	21	g	77	5.0	0.2	132.0	28.10	98.30	6.31
	1	slice							
Neufchatel	100	g	253	9.2	3.6	334.0	152.0	138.0	22.78
	28.35	g	72	2.6	1.0	94.7	43.10	39.10	6.46
	1	oz							
Provolone	100	g	351	25.6	2.1	727.0	138.0	496.0	26.62
	21	g	74	5.4	0.4	153.0	29.00	104.0	5.59
	1	slice							
Romano	100	g	387	31.8	3.6	1433.0	86.00	760.0	26.94
	28.35	g	110	9.0	1.0	406.0	24.40	215.0	7.64
	1	oz							
Swiss	100	g	393	27.0	1.4	185.0	71.00	574.0	31.00
	21	g	83	5.7	0.3	38.8	14.90	121.0	6.51
	1	slice							
Tilsiter/ Tilsit	100	g	340	24.4	1.9	753.0	65.00	500.0	25.98
	28.35	g	96	6.9	0.5	213.0	18.40	142.0	7.36
	1	oz							

CREAM	SERVING QUANTITY	SERVING UNIT	CALORIES (kcal)	PROTEIN (g)	TOTAL CARBOHYDRATES (g)	SODIUM (mg)	POTASSIUM (mg)	PHOSPHORUS (mg)	TOTAL FAT (g)
sour cream, regular	100	g	198	2.4	4.6	31.0	125.00	76.00	19.35
	30 1	g container	59	0.7	1.4	9.3	37.50	22.80	5.80
sour cream, light	100	g	136	3.5	7.1	83.0	212.00	71.00	10.60
	240 1	g cup	326	8.4	17.0	199.0	509.00	170.0	25.40
sour cream, imitation	100	g	208	2.4	6.6	102.0	161.00	45.00	19.52
	240 1	g cup	499	5.8	15.9	245.0	386.00	108.0	46.80
sour cream, fat free	100	g	74	3.1	15.6	141.0	129.00	95.00	0.00
	240 1	g cup	178	7.4	37.4	338.0	310.00	228.0	0.00
heavy full cream	100	g	340	2.8	2.8	27.0	95.00	58.00	36.08
	30 1	g fl oz	102	0.9	1.0	8.1	28.50	17.40	10.80
whipped	100	g	343	2.7	8.6	26.0	89.00	55.00	33.94
	40 1	g cup	137	1.1	3.4	10.4	35.60	22.00	13.60
half and half	100	g	131	3.1	4.3	61.0	132.00	95.00	11.50
	30 1	g fl oz	39	0.9	1.3	18.3	39.60	28.50	3.45
coffee, light cream	100	g	195	3.0	3.7	72.0	136.00	92.00	19.10
	11 1	g ind. container	21	0.3	0.4	7.9	15.00	10.10	2.10

93

D. Fats

(Oils, Nuts, & Seeds)

Hey there!

Do you need to print out this Food List?

You can download a printable version of this chart by scanning the QR code below or copying the link on your computer browser.

https://go.renaltracker.com/printfoodlist

ALMOND	SERVING QUANTITY	SERVING UNIT	CALORIES (kcal)	PROTEIN (g)	TOTAL CARBOHYDRATES (g)	SODIUM (mg)	POTASSIUM (mg)	PHOSPHORUS (mg)	TOTAL FAT (g)
whole	100	g	579	21.2	21.6	1.00	733.00	481.00	49.9
	35.75	g	207	7.6	7.7	0.36	262.05	171.96	17.9
	0.25	c							
slivered	100	g	579	21.2	21.6	1.00	733.00	481.00	49.9
	27	g	156	5.7	5.8	0.27	197.91	129.87	13.5
	0.25	c							
ground	100	g	579	21.2	21.6	1.00	733.00	481.00	49.9
	23.75	g	138	5.0	5.1	0.24	174.09	114.42	11.9
	0.25	c							
paste (marzipan)	100	g	458	9.0	47.8	9.00	314.00	258.00	27.7
	28.38	g	130	2.6	13.6	2.55	89.10	73.21	7.9
	2	tbsp							
oil	100	g	884	0.0	0.0	0.00	0.00	0.00	100
	13.6	g	120	0.0	0.0	0.00	0.00	0.00	13.6
	1	tbsp							
butter, without salt added	100	g	614	21.0	18.8	227.0	748.00	508.00	55.5
	16	g	98	3.4	3.0	1.12	119.68	81.28	8.9
	1	tbsp							
dry roasted, without salt added	100	g	598	3.0	21.0	3.00	713.00	471.00	52.5
	34.5	g	206	7.2	7.3	1.04	245.99	162.50	18.1
	0.25	c							
oil roasted, without salt	100	g	607	21.2	17.7	1.00	699.00	466.00	55.2
	39.25	g	238	8.3	6.9	0.39	274.36	182.91	21.7
	0.25	c							
milk, unsweetened, shelf stable	100	g	15	0.4	1.3	72.00	67.00	9.00	1.0
	262	g	39	1.1	3.4	188.6	175.54	23.58	2.5
	1	c							
milk, sweetened, vanilla flavor ready-to-drink	100	g	38	0.4	6.6	63.00	50.00	8.00	1.0
	240	g	91	1.0	15.8	151.2	120.00	19.20	2.5
	1	c							
milk, chocolate flavor, unsweetened fortified Vit. D2 and E	100	g	21	0.8	1.3	75.00	96.00	17.00	1.5
	240	g	50	2.0	3.0	180.0	130.40	40.80	3.5
	1	c							

95

WALNUT	SERVING QUANTITY	SERVING UNIT	CALORIES (kCal)	PROTEIN (g)	TOTAL CARBOHYDRATES (g)	SODIUM (mg)	POTASSIUM (mg)	PHOSPHORUS (mg)	TOTAL FAT (g)
english, halves	100	g	654	15.2	13.7	2.00	441.00	346.0	65.2
	25	g	164	3.8	3.4	0.50	110.25	86.50	16.3
	0.25	c							
english, ground	100	g	654	15.2	13.7	2.00	441.00	346.0	65.2
	20	g	131	3.1	2.7	0.40	88.20	69.20	13.0
	0.25	c							
english, chopped	100	g	654	15.2	13.7	2.00	441.00	346.0	65.2
	29.25	g	191	4.5	4.0	0.59	128.99	101.2	19.1
	0.25	c							
butternut or white walnut, dried	100	g	612	24.9	12.1	1.00	421.00	446.0	57.0
	120	g	734	29.9	14.5	1.20	505.20	535.2	68.4
	1	c							
black or american, dried, chopped	100	g	619	24.1	9.6	2.00	523.00	513.0	59.3
	31.25	g	193	7.5	3.0	0.63	163.44	160.3	18.5
	0.25	c							
black or american, dried, ground	100	g	604	23.5	9.3	1.95	509.92	500.2	57.9
	26.67	g	161	6.3	2.5	0.52	135.98	133.4	15.4
	0.33	c							
glazed	100	g	500	8.3	47.6	446.0	232.00	na	35.7
	28.35	g	142	2.4	13.5	126.5	65.77	na	10.1
	1	oz							
oil	100	g	884	0.0	0.0	0.0	0.00	0.00	100.0
	13.6	g	120	0.0	0.0	0.0	0.00	0.00	13.6
	1	tbsp							

PINE

	SERVING QUANTITY	SERVING UNIT	CALORIES (kcal)	PROTEIN (g)	TOTAL CARBOHYDRATES (g)	SODIUM (mg)	POTASSIUM (mg)	PHOSPHORUS (mg)	TOTAL FAT (g)
(Pinyon), dried	100	g	629	11.6	19.3	72.00	628.00	35.00	61.0
	28.35	g	178	3.3	5.5	20.41	178.04	9.92	17.3
	1	oz							
(Pignolia), dried	100	g	673	13.7	13.1	2.00	597.00	575.0	68.4
	8.6	g	58	1.2	1.1	0.17	51.34	49.45	5.9
	1	tbsp							

CHESTNUT

	SERVING QUANTITY	SERVING UNIT	CALORIES (kcal)	PROTEIN (g)	TOTAL CARBOHYDRATES (g)	SODIUM (mg)	POTASSIUM (mg)	PHOSPHORUS (mg)	TOTAL FAT (g)
Japanese	100	g	154	2.3	34.9	14.00	329.00	72.00	0.5
	28.35	g	44	0.6	9.9	3.97	93.27	20.41	0.2
	1	oz							
Chinese	100	g	224	4.2	49.1	3.00	447.00	96.00	1.1
	28.35	g	64	1.2	13.9	0.85	126.72	27.22	0.3
	1	oz							
European, unpeeled	100	g	213	2.4	45.5	3.00	518.00	93.00	2.3
	36.25	g	77	0.9	16.5	1.09	187.78	33.71	0.8
	0.25	c							
European, peeled	100	g	196	1.6	44.2	2.00	484.00	38.00	1.3
	28.35	g	56	0.5	12.5	0.57	137.21	10.77	0.4
	1	oz							
European, roasted	100	g	245	3.2	53.0	2.00	592.00	107.0	2.2
	28.35	g	69	0.9	15.0	0.57	167.83	30.33	0.6
	1	oz							
Japanese, roasted	100	g	201	3.0	45.1	19.00	427.00	93.00	0.8
	28.35	g	57	0.8	12.8	5.39	121.05	26.37	0.2
	1	oz							
Chinese, roasted	100	g	239	4.5	52.4	4.00	477.00	102.0	1.2
	28.35	g	68	1.3	14.8	1.13	135.23	28.92	0.3
	1	oz							
Chinese, boiled and steamed	100	g	153	2.9	33.6	2.00	306.00	66.00	0.8
	28.35	g	43	0.8	9.5	0.57	86.75	18.71	0.2
	1	oz							
European, boiled and steamed	100	g	131	2.0	27.8	27.00	715.00	99.00	1.4
	28.35	g	37	0.6	7.9	7.65	202.70	15.31	0.4
	1	oz							
Japanese, boiled and steamed	100	g	56	0.8	12.6	5.00	119.00	26.00	0.2
	28.35	g	16	0.2	3.6	1.42	33.74	7.37	0.1
	1	oz							

PEANUT	SERVING QUANTITY	SERVING UNIT	CALORIES (kcal)	PROTEIN (g)	TOTAL CARBOHYDRATES (g)	SODIUM (mg)	POTASSIUM (mg)	PHOSPHORUS (mg)	TOTAL FAT (g)
oil	100	g	884	0.0	0.0	0.00	0.00	0.00	100
	13.5	g	119	0.0	0.0	0.00	0.00	0.00	13.5
	1	tbsp							
all types	100	g	567	25.8	16.1	18.00	705.00	376.00	49.2
	36.5	g	207	9.4	5.9	6.57	257.33	137.24	18.0
	0.25	c							
all types, dry roasted, no salt added	100	g	587	24.4	21.4	6.00	634.00	363.00	49.7
(1 oz = 28.35g)	36.5	g	214	8.9	7.8	2.19	231.41	132.50	18.1
	0.25	c							
all types, oil roasted, no salt	100	g	599	28.0	15.3	6.00	726.00	397.00	52.5
	133	g	797	37.3	20.3	7.98	965.58	528.01	69.8
	1	c							
butter, smooth, reduced fat	100	g	520	25.9	36.7	540.0	669.00	369.00	34.0
	36	g	187	9.3	12.8	194.4	240.84	132.84	12.2
	2	tbsp							
butter, smooth, no salt added	100	g	598	22.2	22.3	17.00	558.00	335.00	51.4
	32	g	191	7.1	7.1	5.44	178.56	107.20	16.4
	2	tbsp							
butter, chunky, no salt added	100	g	589	24.1	21.6	17.00	745.00	319.00	49.9
	32	g	188	7.7	6.9	5.44	238.40	102.08	16.0
	2	tbsp							
butter, reduced sodium	100	g	590	24.0	21.8	203.0	747.00	317.00	49.9
	16	g	94	3.8	3.5	32.48	119.52	50.72	8.0
	1	tbsp							
sauce, made with PB, water & soy sauce	100	g	257	6.3	22.0	1338	235.00	107.00	16.0
	18	g	46	1.1	4.0	240.8	42.30	19.26	2.9
	1	tbsp							
brittle	100	g	486	7.6	71.2	445.0	168.00	106.00	19.0
	42.53	g	207	3.2	30.3	189.2	71.44	45.08	8.1
	1.5	oz							
flour, defatted	100	g	327	52.2	34.7	180.0	1,290	760.00	0.6
	30	g	98	15.7	10.4	54.00	387.00	228.00	0.2
	0.5	c							

	SERVING QUANTITY	SERVING UNIT	CALORIES (kcal)	PROTEIN (g)	TOTAL CARBOHYDRATES (g)	SODIUM (mg)	POTASSIUM (mg)	PHOSPHORUS (mg)	TOTAL FAT (g)
CASHEW									
raw	100	g	553	18.2	30.2	12.00	660.00	593.0	43.9
	28.35	g	157	5.2	8.6	3.40	187.11	168.1	12.4
	1	oz							
oil roasted, no salt added	100	g	580	16.8	29.9	13.00	632.00	531.0	47.8
	129	g	748	21.7	38.5	16.77	815.28	685	61.6
	1	c							
dry roasted, no salt aded (halves and whole)	100	g	574	15.3	32.7	16.00	565.00	490.0	46.4
	137	g	786	21.0	44.8	21.92	774.05	671.3	63.5
	1	c							
butter, without salt added	100	g	587	17.6	27.6	15.00	546.00	457.0	49.4
	32	g	188	5.6	8.8	4.80	174.72	146.3	15.8
	2	tbsp							
HAZELNUT									
oil	100	g	884	0.0	0.0	0.00	0.00	0.00	100.0
	13.6	g	120	0.0	0.0	0.00	0.00	0.00	13.6
	1	tbsp							
whole (1 oz= 21 kernels)	100	g	628	15.0	16.7	0.00	680.00	290.0	60.8
	33.75	g	212	5.1	5.6	0.00	229.50	97.88	20.5
	0.25	c							
blanched	100	g	629	13.7	17.0	0.00	658.00	310.0	61.2
	28.35	g	178	3.9	4.8	0.00	186.54	87.89	17.3
	1	oz							
chopped	100	g	628	15.0	16.7	0.00	680.00	290.0	60.8
	28.75	g	181	4.3	4.8	0.00	195.50	83.38	17.5
	0.25	c							
ground	100	g	628	15.0	16.7	0.00	680.00	290.0	60.8
	18.75	g	118	2.8	3.1	0.00	127.50	54.38	11.4
	0.25	c							
dry roasted, without salt added	100	g	646	15.0	17.6	0.00	755.00	310.0	62.4
	28.35	g	183	4.3	5.0	0.00	214.04	87.89	17.7
	1	oz							
spread, chocolate flavored	100	g	539	5.4	62.4	41.00	407.00	152.0	29.7

PECANS	SERVING QUANTITY	SERVING UNIT	CALORIES (kcal)	PROTEIN (g)	TOTAL CARBOHYDRATES (g)	SODIUM (mg)	POTASSIUM (mg)	PHOSPHORUS (mg)	TOTAL FAT (g)
chopped	100	g	691	9.2	13.9	0.00	410.00	277.00	72.0
	109	g	753	10.0	15.1	0.00	446.90	410.00	78.5
	1	c							
halves	100	g	691	9.2	13.9	0.00	410.00	277.00	72.0
	24.75	g	171	2.3	3.4	0.00	101.48	68.56	17.8
	0.25	c							
halves, oil roasted	100	g	715	9.2	13.0	1.00	392.00	263.00	75.2
	110	g	787	10.1	14.3	1.10	431.20	289.30	82.8
	1	c							
dry roasted, without salt added	100	g	710	9.5	13.6	1.00	424.00	293.00	74.3
	28.35	g	201	2.7	3.8	0.28	120.20	83.07	21.1
	1	oz							
PISTACHIO									
raw	100	g	560	20.2	27.2	1.00	1,025	490.00	45.3
(1 oz = 49 kernels)	123	g	689	24.8	33.4	1.23	1,261	602.70	55.7
	1	c							
dry roasted, no salt added	100	g	572	21.1	28.3	6.00	1,007	469.00	45.8
	123	g	704	25.9	34.8	7.38	1,239	576.87	56.4
	1	c							
MACADAMIA									
whole or halves	100	g	718	7.9	13.8	5.00	368.00	188.00	75.8
(1 oz = 10-12 kernels)	134	g	962	10.6	18.5	6.70	493.12	251.92	101.5
	1	c							
dry roasted, without salt added	100	g	718	7.8	13.4	4.00	363.00	198.00	76.1
	33.5	g	241	2.6	4.5	1.34	121.61	66.33	25.5
	0.25	c							

SESAME

	SERVING QUANTITY	SERVING UNIT	CALORIES (kcal)	PROTEIN (g)	TOTAL CARBOHYDRATES (g)	SODIUM (mg)	POTASSIUM (mg)	PHOSPHORUS (mg)	TOTAL FAT (g)
seeds, kernels,	100	g	567	17.0	26.0	39.00	406.00	774.00	48.0
toasted	128	g	726	21.7	33.3	49.92	519.68	990.72	61.4
	1	c							
butter or Tahini	100	g	592	17.4	21.5	35.00	459.00	790.00	53.0
	30	g	178	5.2	6.5	10.50	137.70	237.00	15.9
	2	tbsp							
seeds, whole,	100	g	573	17.7	23.5	11.00	468.00	629.00	49.7
dried	9	g	52	1.6	2.1	0.99	42.12	56.61	4.5
	1	tbsp							
butter or Tahini, from	100	g	595	17.0	21.2	115.00	414.00	732.00	53.8
roasted/toasted kernels	30	g	179	5.1	6.4	34.50	124.20	219.60	16.1
	2	tbsp							
SUNFLOWER									
seeds, kernels,	100	g	619	17.2	20.6	3.00	491.00	1,158	56.8
toasted	33.5	g	207	5.8	6.9	1.01	164.49	387.93	19.0
	0.25	c							
seeds, kernels,	100	g	584	20.8	20.0	9.00	645.00	660.00	51.5
dried	36	g	210	7.5	7.2	3.24	232.20	237.60	18.5
	0.25	c							
seeds, kernels,	100	g	592	20.1	22.9	3.00	483.00	1,139	51.3
oil roasted	135	g	799	27.1	31.0	4.05	652.05	1,538	69.3
	1	c							
seeds, kernel.	100	g	582	19.3	24.1	3.00	850.00	1,155	49.8
dry roasted	32	g	186	6.2	7.7	0.96	272.00	369.60	15.9
	0.25	c							
butter, without	100	g	617	17.3	23.3	3.00	576.00	666.00	55.2
salt added	16	g	99	2.8	3.7	0.48	92.16	106.56	8.8
	1	tbsp							
oil, <60% / >60%/	100	g	884	0.0	0.0	0.00	0.00	0.00	100
>70% Linoleic	13.6	g	120	0.0	0.0	0.00	0.00	0.00	13.6
	1	tbsp							
oil, industrial, mid-oleic	100	g	884	0.0	0.0	0.00	0.00	0.00	100
for frying and salad dressings	13.6	g	120	0.0	0.0	0.00	0.00	0.00	13.6
	1	tbsp							

ACORN

	SERVING QUANTITY	SERVING UNIT	CALORIES (kcal)	PROTEIN (g)	TOTAL CARBOHYDRATES (g)	SODIUM (mg)	POTASSIUM (mg)	PHOSPHORUS (mg)	TOTAL FAT (g)
Nuts	100	g	387	6.2	40.8	0.00	539.00	79.00	23.9
	28.35	g	110	1.7	11.6	0.00	152.81	22.40	6.8
	1	oz							
flour	100	g	501	7.5	54.7	0.00	712.00	103.0	30.2
	28.35	g	142	2.1	15.5	0.00	201.85	29.20	8.6
	1	oz							
nuts, dried	100	g	509	8.1	53.7	0.00	709.00	103.0	31.4
	28.35	g	144	2.3	15.2	0.00	201.00	29.20	8.9
	1	oz							

CHIA

seeds, dried	100	g	486	16.5	42.1	16.00	407.00	860.0	30.7
	28.35	g	138	4.7	11.9	4.54	115.38	243.8	8.7
	1	oz							

HEMP

seeds, hulled	100	g	553	31.6	8.7	5.00	1,200	1,650	48.8
	30	g	166	9.5	2.6	1.50	360.00	495.0	14.6
	3	tbsp							

FLAXSEED

seeds, whole	100	g	534	18.3	28.9	30.00	813.00	642.0	42.2
	10.3	g	55	1.9	3.0	3.09	83.70	66.10	4.3
	1	tbsp							
seeds, ground	7	g	37	1.3	2.0	2.10	56.90	44.90	3.0
	1	tbsp							
oil	100	g	884	0.1	0.0	0.00	0.00	1.00	100.0
	14	g	124	0.0	0.0	0.00	0.00	0.14	14.0
	1	tbsp							
oil with added sliced flaxseed	100	g	878	0.4	0.4	6.00	31.00	27.00	99.0
	13.7	g	120	0.1	0.1	0.82	4.25	3.70	13.6
	1	tbsp							
oil, cold pressed	100	g	884	0.1	0.0	0.00	0.00	1.00	100.0
	13.6	g	120	0.0	0.0	0.00	0.00	0.14	13.6
	1	tbsp							

PUMPKIN	SERVING QUANTITY	SERVING UNIT	CALORIES (kCal)	PROTEIN (g)	TOTAL CARBOHYDRATES (g)	SODIUM (mg)	POTASSIUM (mg)	PHOSPHORUS (mg)	TOTAL FAT (g)
meat, 1" cubes	100	g	26	1.0	6.5	1.00	340.00	44.00	0.1
	116	g	30	1.2	7.5	1.16	394.40	51.04	0.1
	1	c							
flowers	100	g	15	1.0	3.3	5.00	173.00	49.00	0.1
	33	g	1	0.0	0.1	0.20	6.92	1.96	0.0
	1	c							
meat, boiled, drained, no salt added	100	g	20	0.7	4.9	1.00	230.00	30.00	0.1
	122.5	g	25	0.9	6.0	1.23	281.75	36.75	0.1
	0.5	c							
pumpkin pie spice powder	100	g	342	5.8	69.3	52.00	663.00	118.0	12.6
	1.7	g	6	0.1	1.2	0.88	11.27	2.01	0.2
	1	tsp							
seed sunfish, cooked dry heat	100	g	114	24.9	0.0	103.0	449.00	231.00	0.9
	85.05	g	97	21.2	0.0	87.60	381.87	196.46	0.8
	3	oz							
seeds, kernels, whole, roasted without salt added	100	g	446	18.6	53.8	18.00	919.00	92.00	19.4
	32	g	143	5.9	17.2	5.76	294.08	29.44	6.2
	0.5	c							
POPPYSEED									
oil	100	g	884	0.0	0.0	0.00	0.00	0.00	100
	13.6	g	120	0.0	0.0	0.00	0.00	0.00	13.6
	1	tbsp							
salad dressing, creamy	100	g	399	0.9	23.7	933.0	61.00	49.00	33.3
	33	g	132	0.3	7.8	307.9	20.13	16.17	11.0
	2	tbsp							

OLIVE	SERVING QUANTITY	SERVING UNIT	CALORIES (kcal)	PROTEIN (g)	TOTAL CARBOHYDRATES (g)	SODIUM (mg)	POTASSIUM (mg)	PHOSPHORUS (mg)	TOTAL FAT (g)
oil, extra virgin,	100	g	884	0.0	0.0	2.00	1.00	0.00	100
virgin	14	g	124	0.0	0.0	0.28	0.14	0.00	14.0
	1	tbsp							
black, kalamata	100	g	116	0.8	6.0	735.0	8.00	3.00	10.9
	15	g	17	0.1	0.9	110.0	1.20	0.45	1.6
	3	pcs							
green	100	g	145	1.0	3.8	1556	42.00	4.00	15.3
	15	g	22	0.2	0.6	233	6.30	0.60	2.3
	3	pcs							
spread	100	g	278	0.7	4.2	835	17.00	3.00	30.1
(tapenade)	16	g	45	0.1	0.7	134	2.72	0.48	4.8
	1	tbsp							
stuffed	100	g	128	1.0	4.0	1340	58.00	6.00	13.2
	15	g	19	0.2	0.6	201	8.70	0.90	2.0
	3	pcs							
COCONUT									
fresh	100	g	354	3.3	15.2	20.00	356.00	113.00	33.5
	85	g	301	2.8	12.9	17.00	303.00	96.00	28.5
	1	c							
water,	100	g	18	0.2	4.2	26.00	165.00	5.00	0.0
unsweetened	240	g	43	0.5	10.2	62.40	396.00	12.00	0.0
	1	c							
milk	100	g	31	0.2	2.9	19.00	19.00	0.00	2.1
	244	g	76	0.5	7.1	46.40	46.40	0.00	5.1
	1	c							
milk/cream **for**	100	g	230	2.3	5.5	15.00	263.00	100.00	23.8
cooking	240	g	552	5.5	13.3	36.00	631.00	240.00	57.2
	1	c							
yogurt	100	g	64	0.3	8.0	21.00	27.00	2.00	3.5
	170	g	109	0.5	13.5	35.70	45.90	3.40	6.0
	6	oz							
cream, canned,	100	g	357	1.2	53.2	36.00	101.00	22.00	16.3
sweetened	37	g	132	0.4	19.7	13.30	37.40	8.14	6.0
	1/4	c							
oil	100	g	833	0.0	0.0	0.00	0.00	0.00	99.1
	14	g	117	0.0	0.0	0.00	0.00	0.00	13.9
	1	tbsp							
flaked, shredded,	100	g	456	3.1	51.9	285.00	361.00	100.00	28.0
packed	28	g	128	1.0	14.5	79.80	101.00	28.00	7.8
	2	tbsp							

	SERVING QUANTITY	SERVING UNIT	CALORIES (kcal)	PROTEIN (g)	TOTAL CARBOHYDRATES (g)	SODIUM (mg)	POTASSIUM (mg)	PHOSPHORUS (mg)	TOTAL FAT (g)
SAFFLOWER									
oil	100	g	884	0.0	0.0	0.00	0.00	0.00	100.0
	14	g	124	0.0	0.0	0.00	0.00	0.00	14.0
	1	tbsp							
CANOLA									
oil	100	g	884	0.0	0.0	0.00	0.00	0.00	100.0
	14	g	124	0.0	0.0	0.00	0.00	0.00	14.0
	1	tbsp							
SOYBEAN									
oil	100	g	884	0.0	0.0	0.00	0.00	0.00	100.0
	14	g	124	0.0	0.0	0.00	0.00	0.00	14.0
	1	tbsp							
BUTTER									
stick	100	g	717	0.9	0.1	643.00	24.00	24.00	81.1
	14	g	100	0.1	0.0	90.00	3.36	3.36	11.4
	1	tbsp							
light, stick or tub	100	g	499	3.3	0.0	450.00	71.00	34.00	55.1
	14	g	70	0.5	0.0	63.00	9.94	4.76	7.7
	1	tbsp							
unsalted	100	g	717	0.9	0.1	11.00	24.00	24.00	81.1
	14	g	102	0.1	0.0	1.56	3.41	3.41	11.5
	1	tbsp							
GHEE									
clarified butter	100	g	876	0.3	0.0	2.00	5.00	3.00	99.5
	14	g	123	0.0	0.0	0.28	0.70	0.42	13.9
	1	tbsp							
MARGARINE									
stick	100	g	717	0.2	0.7	751.00	18.00	5.00	80.7
	14	g	100	0.0	0.1	105.00	2.52	0.70	11.3
	1	tbsp							

E. Vegetables

Hey there!

Do you need to print out this Food List?

You can download a printable version of this chart by scanning the QR code below or copying the link on your computer browser.

https://go.renaltracker.com/printfoodlist

TOMATO	SERVING QUANTITY	SERVING UNIT	CALORIES (kcal)	PROTEIN (g)	TOTAL CARBOHYDRATES (g)	SODIUM (mg)	POTASSIUM (mg)	PHOSPHORUS (mg)	TOTAL FAT (g)
red, whole	100.00	g	18	0.9	3.9	5.00	237	24.00	
medium 2.6 in	123.00	g	22	1.1	4.8	6.15	292	29.52	
diameter	1.00	pc							
diced or	100.00	g	18	0.9	3.9	5.00	237	24.00	
chopped	90.00	g	16	0.8	3.5	4.50	213	21.60	
	0.50	c							
yellow, chopped	100.00	g	15	1.0	3.0	23.00	258	36.00	
	92.67	g	14	0.9	2.8	21.31	239	33.36	
	0.67	c							
orange,	100.00	g	16	1.2	3.2	42.00	212	29.00	
chopped	79.00	g	13	0.9	2.5	33.18	167	22.91	
	0.50	c							
green	100.00	g	23	1.2	5.1	13.00	204	28.00	
	90.00	g	21	1.1	4.6	11.70	183	25.20	
	0.50	c							
whole, canned	100.00	g	16	0.8	3.5	115	191	17.00	
	240.00	g	38	1.9	8.3	276	458	40.80	
	1.00	c							
sauce, canned,	100.00	g	24	1.2	5.3	11.00	297	27.00	
no salt	244.00	g	59	2.9	13.0	26.84	725	65.88	
	1.00	c							
crushed, canned	100.00	g	32	1.6	7.3	186	293	32.00	
	56.70	g	18	0.9	4.1	106	166	18.14	
	2.00	oz							
paste, canned	100.00	g	82	4.3	18.9	790	1,014	83.00	
	32.80	g	27	1.4	6.2	259	333	27.22	
	2.00	tbsp							
puree, canned,	100.00	g	38	1.7	9.0	28.00	439	40.00	
no salt	250.00	g	95	4.1	22.5	70.00	1,098	100.00	
	1.00	c							
sun dried, in oil,	100.00	g	213	5.1	23.3	266	1,565	139.00	
drained	27.50	g	59	1.4	6.4	73.15	430	38.23	
	0.25	c							
Ketchup, low	100.00	g	101	1.0	27.4	20.00	281	26.00	
sodium	15.00	g	15	0.2	4.1	3.00	42.15	3.90	
	1.00	tbsp							
juice, canned	100.00	g	17	0.9	3.5	253	217	19.00	
	243.00	g	41	2.1	8.6	614	527	46.17	
	8.00	fl oz							
cherry, sweet,	100.00	g	63	1.1	16.0	0.00	222	21.00	
raw	138.00	g	87	1.5	22.1	0.00	306	29.00	
	1.00	c							

ASPARAGUS	SERVING QUANTITY	SERVING UNIT	CALORIES (kCal)	PROTEIN (g)	TOTAL CARBOHYDRATES (g)	SODIUM (mg)	POTASSIUM (mg)	PHOSPHORUS (mg)	TOTAL FAT (g)
boiled,	100.00	g	22	2.4	4.1	14.00	224.00	54.00	0.22
drained	90.00	g	20	2.2	3.7	12.60	201.60	48.60	0.20
	0.50	c							
frozen	100.00	g	24	3.2	4.1	8.00	253.00	64.00	0.23
	87.00	g	21	2.8	3.6	6.96	220.11	55.68	0.20
	6.00	pcs							
frozen,	100.00	g	18	3.0	1.9	3.00	172.00	49.00	0.42
boiled, drained	90.00	g	16	2.7	1.7	2.70	154.80	44.10	0.38
	0.50	c							
canned,	100.00	g	19	2.1	2.5	287.00	172.00	43.00	0.65
drained	121.00	g	23	2.6	3.0	347.27	208.12	52.03	0.79
	0.50	c							
BEANS									
green wax,	100.00	g	31	1.8	7.0	6.00	211.00	38.00	
raw	82.50	g	26	1.5	5.8	4.95	174.08	31.35	
	0.75	c							
green wax,	100.00	g	33	1.8	7.5	3.00	186.00	32.00	
frozen	82.67	g	27	1.5	6.2	2.48	153.76	26.45	
	0.67	c							
green wax,	100.00	g	35	1.9	7.9	1.00	146.00	29.00	
boiled, drained	125.00	g	44	2.4	9.9	1.25	182.50	36.25	
	1.00	c							
green wax,	100.00	g	21	1.1	4.2	268.00	96.00	22.00	
canned,	135.00	g	28	1.4	5.7	361.80	129.60	29.70	
drained	1.00	c							
CARROTS									
strips, slices	100.00	g	41	0.9	9.6	69.00	320.00	35.00	
	122.00	g	50	1.1	11.7	84.18	390.40	42.70	
	1.00	c							
grated	100.00	g	41	0.9	9.6	69.00	320.00	35.00	
	82.50	g	34	0.8	7.9	56.93	264.00	28.88	
	0.75	c							
sliced, boiledd rained, no salt	100.00	g	35	0.8	8.2	58.00	235.00	30.00	
	78.00	g	27	0.6	6.4	45.24	183.30	23.40	
	0.50	c							
frozen	100.00	g	36	0.8	7.9	68.00	235.00	33.00	
	85.33	g	31	0.7	6.7	58.03	200.53	28.16	
	0.67	c							
baby	100.00	g	35	0.6	8.2	78.00	237.00	28.00	
	80.00	g	28	0.5	6.6	62.40	189.60	22.40	
	8.00	pcs							
juice, canned	100.00	g	40	1.0	9.3	66.00	292.00	42.00	
	236.00	g	94	2.2	21.9	155.76	689.12	99.12	
	8.00	fl oz							

CORN	SERVING QUANTITY	SERVING UNIT	CALORIES (kcal)	PROTEIN (g)	TOTAL CARBOHYDRATES (g)	SODIUM (mg)	POTASSIUM (mg)	PHOSPHORUS (mg)	TOTAL FAT (g)
white, sweet	100.00	g	390	7.8	86.6	956.00	88.00	39.00	
	25.00	g	98	2.0	21.7	239.00	22.00	9.75	
	1.00	c							
white, steamed (Navajo)	100.00	g	386	9.7	75.2	4.00	532.00	312.00	
	85.05	g	328	8.3	64.0	3.40	452.47	265.36	
	3.00	oz							
white, stew, steamed (Navajo)	100.00	g	112	8.8	10.8	104.00	177.00	107.00	
	85.05	g	95	7.5	9.2	88.45	150.54	91.00	
	3.00	oz							
sweet, boiled, drained	100.00	g	94	3.1	22.3	4.00	251.00	75.00	0.74
	82.00	g	77	2.6	18.3	3.28	205.82	61.50	0.61
	0.50	c							
flour, white, whole grain	100.00	g	361	6.9	76.9	5.00	315.00	272.00	3.86
	29.25	g	106	2.0	22.5	1.46	92.14	79.56	1.13
	0.25	c							
yellow, sweet, boiled, drained	100.00	g	96	3.4	21.0	1.00	218.00	77.00	1.50
	82.00	g	79	2.8	17.2	0.82	178.76	63.14	1.23
	0.50	c							
yellow, sweet, on the cob	100.00	g	86	3.3	18.7	15.00	270.00	89.00	1.35
	154.00	g	77	2.9	16.8	13.50	243.00	80.10	1.22
	1.00	c							
yello, sweet, creamed, canned	100.00	g	72	1.7	18.1	261.00	134.00	51.00	0.42
	128.00	g	92	2.2	23.2	334.08	171.52	65.28	0.54
	0.50	c							
yellow, sweet, kernels, frozen	100.00	g	88	3.0	20.7	3.00	213.00	70.00	0.78
	82.00	g	72	2.5	17.0	2.46	174.66	57.40	0.64
	0.50	c							
yellow, sweet, canned with liquid	100.00	g	61	2.0	13.9	195.00	136.00	46.00	0.77
	128.00	g	78	2.5	17.7	249.60	174.08	58.88	0.99
	0.50	c							
tortilla, no salt added	100.00	g	222	5.7	46.6	11.00	154.00	314.00	2.50
	26.00	g	58	1.5	12.1	2.86	40.04	81.64	0.65
	1.00	pc							

MUSH ROOM	SERVING QUANTITY	SERVING UNIT	CALORIES (kcal)	PROTEIN (g)	TOTAL CARBOHYDRATES (g)	SODIUM (mg)	POTASSIUM (mg)	PHOSPHORUS (mg)	TOTAL FAT (g)
Shitake, raw	100.00	g	34	2.2	6.8	9.00	304	112.00	
	19.00	g	6	0.4	1.3	1.71	57.76	21.28	
	1.00	pc							
Shitake, dried	100.00	g	296	9.6	75.4	13.00	1,534	294.00	
	32.40	g	96	3.1	24.4	4.21	497	95.26	
	9.00	pcs							
Shitake, cooked	100.00	g	56	1.6	14.4	4.00	117	29.00	
	72.50	g	41	1.1	10.4	2.90	84.83	21.03	
	0.50	c							
Shitake, stir fried	100.00	g	39	3.5	7.7	5.00	326	111.00	
	108.00	g	42	3.7	8.3	5.40	352	119.88	
	1.00	c							
Portabella/ Portabello	100.00	9	22	2.1	3.9	9.00	364	108.00	
Portabello, grilled	100.00	g	29	3.3	4.4	11.00	437	135.00	
White, raw	100.00	g	22	3.0	3.3	5.00	318	86.00	
	96.00	g	21	3.0	3.1	4.80	305	82.56	
	1.00	c							
white, sliced, stir-fried	100.00	g	26	3.6	4.0	12.00	396	105.00	
	108.00	g	28	3.9	4.4	12.96	428	113.40	
	1.00	c							

LETTUCE

LETTUCE	SERVING QUANTITY	SERVING UNIT	CALORIES (kcal)	PROTEIN (g)	TOTAL CARBOHYDRATES (g)	SODIUM (mg)	POTASSIUM (mg)	PHOSPHORUS (mg)	TOTAL FAT (g)
romaine, shredded	100.00	g	17	1.2	3.3	8.00	247.00	30.0	
	70.50	g	12	0.9	2.3	5.64	174.14	21.1	
	1.50	c							
butterhead, medium leaves	100.00	g	13	1.4	2.2	5.00	238.00	33.0	
	82.50	g	11	1.1	1.8	4.13	196.35	27.2	
	11.00	pcs							
Red Leaf, shredded	100.00	g	13	1.3	2.3	25	187	28.00	
	28.00	g	4	0.4	0.6	7	52.36	7.84	
	1.00	c							
Iceberg, shredded or chopped	100.00	g	14	0.9	3.0	10	141	20.00	
	108.00	g	15	1.0	3.2	11	152.28	21.60	
	1.50	c							
Iceberg, loose leaves, medium	100.00	g	14	0.9	3.0	10	141.00	20.00	
	80.00	g	11	0.7	2.4	8	112.80	16.00	
	10.00	pcs							

CABBAGE

	SERVING QUANTITY	SERVING UNIT	CALORIES (kcal)	PROTEIN (g)	TOTAL CARBOHYDRATES (g)	SODIUM (mg)	POTASSIUM (mg)	PHOSPHORUS (mg)	TOTAL FAT (g)
green, chopped	100.00	g	25	1.3	5.8	18.00	170.00	26.00	
	89.00	g	22	1.1	5.2	16.02	151.30	23.14	
	1.00	c							
green shredded, sliced	100.00	g	25	1.3	5.8	18.00	170.00	26.00	
	87.50	g	22	1.1	5.1	15.75	148.75	22.75	
	1.25	c							
green, shredded, boiled, drained, no salt added	100.00	g	23	1.3	5.5	8.00	196.00	33.00	
	75.00	g	17	1.0	4.1	6.00	147.00	24.75	
	0.50	c							
chinese, shredded, raw	100.00	g							
	76.00	g	12	0.9		6.84	181.00	22.04	
	1.00	c							
chinese, cooked, no salt	100.00	g							
	75.00	g	17	1.0		6.00	147.00	24.75	
	0.50	c							
red, shredded	100.00	g	31	1.4	7.4	27.00	243.00	30.00	
	87.50	g	27	1.3	6.5	23.63	212.63	26.25	
	1.25	c							
red, shredded, boiled, drained, no salt added	100.00	g	29	1.5	6.9	28.00	262.00	33.00	
	75.00	g	27	1.1	5.2	21.00	196.50	24.75	
	0.50	c							
Bok Choy or White Mustard, shredded	100.00	g	13	1.5	2.2	65.00	252.00	37.00	
	87.50	g	11	1.3	1.9	56.88	220.50	32.38	
	1.25	c							
Bok Choy/ Pak Choi, shredded, boiled, drained	100.00	g	12	1.6	1.8	34.00	371.00	29.00	
	85.00	g	10	1.3	1.5	28.90	315.35	24.65	
	0.50	c							
Kimchi	100.00	g	15	1.1	2.4	498.00	151.00	24.00	
	150.00	g	23	1.7	3.6	747.00	226.50	36.00	
	1.00	c							

PEPPER	SERVING QUANTITY	SERVING UNIT	CALORIES (kcal)	PROTEIN (g)	TOTAL CARBOHYDRATES (g)	SODIUM (mg)	POTASSIUM (mg)	PHOSPHORUS (mg)	TOTAL FAT (g)
bell, sweet yellow, 3 in diameter	100.00	g	27	1.0	6.3	2.00	212.00	24.00	
	186.00	g	50	1.9	11.8	3.72	394.32	44.64	
	1.00	pc							
bell, sweet green, chopped	100.00	g	20	0.9	4.6	3.00	175.00	20.00	
	74.50	g	15	0.6	3.5	2.24	130.38	14.90	
	0.50	c							
bell, sweet green, sauteed	100.00	g	116	0.8	4.2	17.00	134.00	15.00	
bell, sweet red, chopped	100.00	g	26	1.0	6.0	4.00	211.00	26.00	
	74.50	g	19	0.7	4.5	2.98	157.20	19.37	
	0.50	c							
bell, sweet red, sauteed	100.00	g	133	1.0	6.6	21.00	193.00	23.00	
bell, sweet red, chopped, frozen, drained, boiled, no salt added	100.00	g	16	1.0	3.3	4.00	72.00	13.00	
	85.05	g	14	0.8	2.8	3.40	61.24	11.06	
	3.00	oz							
jalapeno, sliced	100.00	g	29	0.9	6.5	3.00	248.00	26.00	
	22.50	g	7	0.2	1.5	0.68	55.80	5.85	
	0.13	c							
serrano, chopped	100.00	g	32	1.7	6.7	10.00	305.00	40.00	
	26.25	g	8	0.5	1.8	2.63	80.06	10.50	
	0.25	c							
black, ground	100.00	g	251	10.4	64.0	20.00	1,329.00	158.00	
	2.10	g	5	0.2	1.3	0.42	27.91	3.32	
	1.00	tsp							
white, ground	100.00	g	296	10.4	68.6	5.00	73.00	176.00	
	2.40	g	7	0.3	1.7	0.12	1.75	4.22	
	1.00	tsp							
hot chilli, red	100.00	g	40	1.9	8.8	9.00	322.00	43.00	
	45.00	g	18	0.8	4.0	4.05	144.90	19.35	
	1.00	pc							

	SERVING QUANTITY	SERVING UNIT	CALORIES (kcal)	PROTEIN (g)	TOTAL CARBOHYDRATES (g)	SODIUM (mg)	POTASSIUM (mg)	PHOSPHORUS (mg)	TOTAL FAT (g)
BROCCOLI									
florets, raw	100.00	g	28	3.0	5.1	27.00	325.00	66.00	0.35
	71.00	g	20	2.1	3.6	19.17	230.75	46.86	0.25
	1.00	c							
Cooked, no salt	100.00	g	35	2.4	7.2	41.00	293.00	67.00	0.41
	78.00	g	27	1.9	5.6	31.98	228.54	52.26	0.32
	0.50	c							
frozen, spears	100.00	g	29	3.1	5.4	17.00	250.00	59.00	0.34
	85.05	g	25	2.6	4.6	14.46	212.62	50.18	0.29
	3.00	oz							
CAULIFLOWER									
green,raw	100.00	g	31	3.0	6.1	23.00	300.00	62.00	0.30
	64.00	g	20	1.9	3.9	14.72	192.00	39.68	0.19
	1.00	c							
cooked, no salt	100.00	g	32	3.0	6.3	23.00	278.00	57.00	0.31
	62.00	g	20	1.9	3.9	14.26	172.36	35.34	0.19
	0.50	c							
CUCUMBER									
sliced, raw	100.00	g	15	0.7	3.6	2.00	147.00	24.00	0.11
	52.00	g	8	0.3	1.9	1.04	76.44	12.48	0.06
	0.50	c							
sliced	100.00	g	15	0.7	3.6	2.00	147.00	24.00	0.11
	78.00	g	12	0.5	2.8	1.56	114.66	18.72	0.09
	0.75	c							
BEETS									
raw	100.00	g	43	1.6	9.6	78.00	325.00	40.00	0.17
	90.67	g	39	1.5	8.7	70.72	294.67	36.27	0.15
	0.67	c							
whole or sliced, boiled, drained, no salt	100.00	g	44	1.7	10.0	77.00	305.00	38.00	0.18
whole, canned	100.00	g	30	0.7	7.1	143.00	159.00	15.00	0.09
	246.00	g	74	1.8	17.6	351.78	391.14	36.90	0.22
	1.00	c							
sliced, canned, drained	100.00	g	31	0.9	7.2	194.00	148.00	17.00	0.14
	85.00	g	26	0.8	6.1	164.90	125.80	14.45	0.12
	0.50	c							

POTATOES	SERVING QUANTITY	SERVING UNIT	CALORIES (kcal)	PROTEIN (g)	TOTAL CARBOHYDRATES (g)	SODIUM (mg)	POTASSIUM (mg)	PHOSPHORUS (mg)	TOTAL FAT (g)
russet, flesh and skin	100.00	g	79	2.1	18.1	5.00	417.00	55.00	0.08
russet, flesh and skin, baked	100.00	g	95	2.6	21.4	14.00	550.00	71.00	0.13
	173.00	g	164	4.6	37.1	24.22	951.50	122.83	0.22
	1.00	pc							
white, flesh and skin	100.00	g	69	1.7	15.7	16.00	407.00	62.00	0.10
white, flesh and skin, baked	100.00	g	92	2.1	21.1	7.00	544.00	75.00	0.15
	173.00	g	159	3.6	36.5	12.11	941.12	129.75	0.26
	1.00	pcs							
french fries, frozen	100.00	g	147	2.2	24.8	332.00	408.00	83.00	4.66
	71.50	g	105	1.6	17.7	237.38	291.72	59.35	3.33
	11.00	pcs							
sweet,cubed	100.00	g	86	1.6	20.1	55.00	337.00	47.00	0.05
	99.75	g	86	1.6	20.1	54.86	336.16	46.88	0.05
	0.75	c							
sweet, boiled, mashed	100.00	g	76	1.4	17.7	27.00	230.00	32.00	0.14
	328.00	g	249	4.5	58.1	88.56	754.40	104.96	0.46
	1.00	c							
sweet, frozen, baked	100.00	g	100	1.7	23.4	8.00	377.00	44.00	0.12
	117.33	g	117	2.0	27.5	9.39	442.35	51.63	0.14
	0.67	c							
sweet, baked, peeled	100.00	g	90	2.0	20.7	36.00	475.00	54.00	0.15
	0.50	c							
chips, unsalted	100.00	g	536	7.0	52.9	8.00	1,275	165.00	34.60
	28.35	g	152	2.0	15.0	2.27	361.46	46.78	9.81
	1.00	oz							
hash browns, frozen	100.00	g	82	2.1	17.7	22.00	285.00	47.00	0.62
	70.00	g	57	1.4	12.4	15.40	199.50	32.90	0.43
	0.33	c							
wedges, frozen	100.00	g	129	2.7	25.5	49.00	394.00	87.00	2.20

PEAS

	SERVING QUANTITY	SERVING UNIT	CALORIES (Kcal)	PROTEIN (g)	TOTAL CARBOHYDRATES (g)	SODIUM (mg)	POTASSIUM (mg)	PHOSPHORUS (mg)	TOTAL FAT (g)
green	100.00	g	81	5.4	14.5	5.00	244.00	108.00	0.40
	72.50	g	59	3.9	10.5	3.63	176.90	78.30	0.29
	0.50	c							
green, frozen	100.00	g	77	5.2	13.6	108.00	153.00	82.00	0.40
	72.00	g	55	3.8	9.8	77.76	110.16	59.04	0.29
	0.50	c							
green, boiled,	100.00	g	84	5.4	15.6	3.00	271.00	117.00	0.22
drained	80.00	g	67	4.3	12.5	2.40	216.80	93.60	0.18
	0.50	c							
green, canned,	100.00	g	68	4.5	11.4	273.00	106.00	67.00	0.80
drained	87.50	g	60	3.9	9.9	238.88	92.75	58.63	0.70
	0.50	c							
green, frozen,	100.00	g	78	5.2	14.3	72.00	110.00	77.00	0.27
boiled, drained	80.00	g	62	4.1	11.4	57.60	88.00	61.60	0.22
	0.50	c							
split, boiled, no	100.00	g	118	8.3	21.1	2.00	362.00	99.00	0.39
salt added	98.00	g	116	8.2	21.0	1.96	354.76	97.02	0.38
	0.50	c							
sugar or snow	100.00	g	42	2.8	7.6	4.00	200.00	53.00	0.20
peas, whole fresh	78.75	g	33	2.2	6.0	3.15	157.50	41.74	0.16
	1.25	c							
snow/sugar,	100.00	g	42	2.8	7.6	4.00	200.00	53.00	0.20
frozen	78.75	g	33	2.2	6.0	3.15	157.50	41.74	0.16
	1.25	c							
snow/sugar,	100.00	g	42	3.3	7.1	4.00	240.00	55.00	0.23
boiled, drained	80.00	g	34	2.6	5.6	3.20	192.00	44.00	0.18
	0.50	c							
snow/sugar,	100.00	g	52	3.5	9.0	5.00	217.00	58.00	0.38
frozen, boiled, drained	80.00	g	42	2.8	7.2	4.00	173.60	46.40	0.30
	0.50	c							

ARTICHOKES	SERVING QUANTITY	SERVING UNIT	CALORIES (kCal)	PROTEIN (g)	TOTAL CARBOHYDRATES (g)	SODIUM (mg)	POTASSIUM (mg)	PHOSPHORUS (mg)	TOTAL FAT (g)
whole, boiled, drained	100.00	g	53	2.9	12.0	60.00	286	73.00	0.34
med size	120.00 1.00	g pc	64	3.5	14.3	72.00	343	87.60	0.41
hearts, boiled, drained	100.00	g	53	2.9	11.9	60.00	286	73.00	0.34
	84.00 0.50	g c	45	2.4	10.0	50.40	240	61.32	0.29
Globe or French, frozen	100.00	g	45	3.1	9.2	53.00	264	61.00	0.50
boiled, drained 1 svg= 1/3 of 9oz package	80.00 1.00	g svg	36	2.5	7.3	42.40	211	48.80	0.40
ALFALFA									
sprouts	100.00	g	23	4.0	2.1	6.00	79.00	70.00	0.69
	33.00 1.00	g c	8	1.3	0.7	1.98	26.07	23.10	0.23
CELERY									
stalk	100.00	g	14	0.7	3.0	80.00	260	24.00	0.17
medium 7.5 - 8 in long	80.00	g	11	0.6	2.4	64.00	208	19.20	0.14
	2.00	stalks							
diced, chopped	100.00	g	14	0.7	3.0	80.00	260	24.00	0.17
	101.00 1.00	g c	14	0.7	3.0	80.80	263	24.24	0.17
celeriac or celery root	100.00	g	42	1.5	9.2	100.00	300	115	0.30
	78.00 0.50	g c	33	1.2	7.2	78.00	234	90	0.23
seeds	100.00	g	392	18.1	41.4	160.00	1,400	547	25.27
	2.00 1.00	g tsp	8	0.4	0.8	3.20	28.00	10.94	0.51
flakes, dried	100.00	g	319	11.3	68.7	1,435.00	4,388	402	2.10
	28.35 1.00	g oz	90	3.2	18.1	406.82	1,244	114	0.60

	SERVING QUANTITY	SERVING UNIT	CALORIES (kcal)	PROTEIN (g)	TOTAL CARBOHYDRATES (g)	SODIUM (mg)	POTASSIUM (mg)	PHOSPHORUS (mg)	TOTAL FAT (g)
COLLARDS									
chopped, raw	100.00	g	32	3.0	5.4	17.00	213.00	25.00	0.61
	90.00	g	29	2.7	4.9	15.30	191.70	22.50	0.55
	2.50	c							
boiled, drained	100.00	g	33	2.7	5.7	15.00	117.00	32.00	0.72
	95.00	g	31	2.6	5.4	14.25	111.15	30.40	0.68
	0.50	c							
frozen, chopped, raw	100.00	g	33	2.7	6.5	48.00	253.00	27.00	0.37
	85.05	g	28	2.3	5.5	40.82	215.17	22.96	0.31
	3.00	oz							
frozen, chopped, boiled/ drained	100.00	g	36	3.0	7.1	50.00	251.00	27.00	0.41
	85.00	g	31	2.5	6.0	42.50	213.35	22.95	0.35
	0.50	c							
EGGPLANT/AUBERGINE									
boiled, drained, no salt cut in 1" cubes	100.00	g	35	0.8	8.7	1.00	123.00	15.00	0.23
	99.00	g	35	0.8	8.6	0.99	121.77	14.85	0.23
	1.00	c							
pickled	100.00	g	49	0.9	9.8	1,674	12.00	9.00	0.70
	136	g	67	1.2	13.3	2,276	16.32	12.24	0.95
	1.00	c							
JICAMA (YAMBEAN)									
raw	100.00	g	38	0.7	8.8	4.00	150.00	18.00	0.09
	86.67	g	33	0.6	7.6	3.47	130.00	15.60	0.08
	0.67	c							
boiled, drained, no salt 1 svg= 3oz	100.00	g	38	0.7	8.8	4.00	135.00	16.00	0.09
	85.05	g	32	0.6	7.5	3.40	114.82	13.61	0.08
	3.00	oz							

ARUGULA	SERVING QUANTITY	SERVING UNIT	CALORIES (kcal)	PROTEIN (g)	TOTAL CARBOHYDRATES (g)	SODIUM (mg)	POTASSIUM (mg)	PHOSPHORUS (mg)	TOTAL FAT (g)
raw, leaves	100	g	25	2.6	3.7	27.00	369	52.00	0.66
	80.00	g	20	2.1	2.9	21.60	295	41.60	0.53
	4.00	c							
salad mixed	100	g	18	1.5	3.3	16.94	299	32.15	0.27
baby greens	41.25	g	7	0.6	1.4	6.99	123	13.26	0.11
Arugula, butterhead, endives, Radicchio	1.00	c							

ENDIVE OR ESCAROLE

	SERVING QUANTITY	SERVING UNIT	CALORIES	PROTEIN	TOTAL CARBOHYDRATES	SODIUM	POTASSIUM	PHOSPHORUS	TOTAL FAT
raw, chopped	100	g	17	1.3	3.4	22.00	314.00	28.00	0.20
	87.50	g	15	1.1	2.9	19.25	274.75	24.50	0.18
	1.75	c							
Chicory, Witlof	100	g	17	0.9	4.0	2.00	211.00	26.00	0.10
or Belgium	90.00	g	15	0.8	3.6	1.80	189.90	23.40	0.09
	1.00	c							

OKRA

	SERVING QUANTITY	SERVING UNIT	CALORIES	PROTEIN	TOTAL CARBOHYDRATES	SODIUM	POTASSIUM	PHOSPHORUS	TOTAL FAT
raw	100	g	33	1.9	7.5	7.00	299.00	61.00	0.19
	75.00	g	25	1.5	5.6	5.25	224.25	45.75	0.14
	0.75	c							
sliced, boiled,	100	g	22	1.9	4.5	6.00	135.00	32.00	0.21
drained, n.s.	80.00	g	18	1.5	3.6	4.80	108.00	25.60	0.17
	0.50	c							
frozen	100	g	30	1.7	6.6	3.00	211.00	42.00	0.25
	85.05	g	26	1.4	5.6	2.55	179.45	35.72	0.21
	3.00	oz							
frozen, boiled,	100	g	29	1.6	6.4	3.00	184.00	37.00	0.24
drained, no salt	92.00	g	27	1.5	5.9	2.76	169.28	34.04	0.22
sliced	0.50	c							

PUMPKIN

	SERVING QUANTITY	SERVING UNIT	CALORIES	PROTEIN	TOTAL CARBOHYDRATES	SODIUM	POTASSIUM	PHOSPHORUS	TOTAL FAT
fruit/meat, raw,	100	g	26	1.0	6.5	1.00	340.00	44.00	0.10
cut 1" cube	116	g	30	1.2	7.5	1.16	394.40	51.04	0.12
	1.00	c							
boiled, drained,	100	g	20	0.7	4.9	1.00	230.00	30.00	0.07
mashed, n.s.	122.5	g	25	0.9	6.0	1.23	281.75	36.75	0.09
	0.50	c							
flowers	100	g	15	0.0	3.3	5.00	173.00	49.00	0.07
	33.00	g	1	0.0	0.1	0.20	6.92	1.96	0.00
	1.00	c							
flowers, boiled,	100	g	15	1.1	3.3	6.00	106.00	34.00	0.08
drained	89.33	g	13	1.0	3.0	5.36	5.36	30.37	0.07
	0.67	c							
seeds (squash	100	g	559	30.2	10.7	7.00	809.00	1,233	49.05
kernels), dried	34.50	g	193	10.4	3.7	2.42	279.11	425.4	16.92
	0.25	c							
seeds	100	g	446	18.6	53.8	18.00	919.00	92.00	19.40
(pumkin/squash),	32.00	g	143	5.9	17.2	5.76	294.08	29.44	6.21
whole, roasted no salt added	0.50	c							

118

SQUASH	SERVING QUANTITY	SERVING UNIT	CALORIES (kcal)	PROTEIN (g)	TOTAL CARBOHYDRATES (g)	SODIUM (mg)	POTASSIUM (mg)	PHOSPHORUS (mg)	TOTAL FAT (g)
winter,	100.00	g	34	1.0	8.6	4.00	350.00	23.00	0.13
all varieties cubes	116.00	g	39	1.1	10.0	4.64	406.00	26.68	0.15
	1.00	c							
butternut	100.00	g	45	1.0	11.7	4.00	352.00	33.00	0.10
cubes	140.00	g	63	1.4	16.4	5.60	492.80	46.20	0.14
	1.00	c							
winter,	100.00	g	57	1.8	14.4	2.00	212.00	22.00	0.10
butternut, frozen	85.05	g	48	1.5	12.3	1.70	180.30	18.71	0.09
	3.00	oz							
summer,	100.00	g	16	1.2	3.4	2.00	262.00	38.00	0.18
all varieties sliced	84.75	g	14	1.0	2.8	1.70	222.05	32.21	0.15
	0.75	c							
KOHLRABI									
raw	100.00	g	27	1.7	6.2	20.00	350.00	46.00	0.10
	135.00	g	36	2.3	8.4	27.00	472.50	62.10	0.14
	1.00	c							
boiled, drained,	100.00	g	29	1.8	6.7	21.00	340.00	45.00	0.11
sliced	165.00	g	48	3.0	11.0	34.65	561.00	74.25	0.18
	1.00	c							
LEEKS									
raw	100.00	g	61	1.5	14.2	20.00	180.00	35.00	0.30
	89.00	g	54	1.3	12.6	17.80	160.20	31.15	0.27
	1.00	c							
boiled, drained,	100.00	g	31	0.8	7.6	10.00	87.00	17.00	0.20
chopped or diced	26.00	g	8	0.2	2.0	2.60	22.62	4.42	0.05
	0.25	c							
CASSAVA/YUCCA/MANIOC									
raw	100.00	g	160	1.4	38.1	14.00	271.00	27.00	0.28
	103.00	g	165	1.4	39.2	14.42	279.13	27.81	0.29
	0.50	c							
RADISH									
oriental (Daikon),	100.00	g	18	0.6	4.1	21.00	227.00	23.00	0.10
7" long	338.00	g	61	2.0	13.9	70.98	767.26	77.74	0.34
	1.00	p c							
oriental, boiled,	100.00	g	17	0.7	3.4	13.00	285.00	24.00	0.24
drained, no salt sliced	73.50	g	13	0.5	2.5	9.56	209.48	17.64	0.18
	0.50	c							
sprouts	100.00	g	43	3.8	3.6	6.00	86.00	113.0	2.53
	38.00	g	16	1.5	1.4	2.28	32.68	42.94	0.96
	1.00	c							

TURNIP GREENS

	SERVING QUANTITY	SERVING UNIT	CALORIES (kcal)	PROTEIN (g)	TOTAL CARBOHYDRATES (g)	SODIUM (mg)	POTASSIUM (mg)	PHOSPHORUS (mg)	TOTAL FAT (g)
raw, turnip	100.00	g	32	1.5	7.1	40.00	296.00	42.00	0.30
greens, chopped	82.50	g	26	1.2	5.9	33.00	244.20	34.65	0.25
	1.50	c							
frozen	100.00	g	22	2.5	3.7	12.00	184.00	27.00	0.31
	82.00	g	18	2.0	3.0	9.84	150.88	22.14	0.25
	0.50	c							
canned	100.00	g	14	1.4	2.4	277.00	141.00	21.00	0.30
	78.00	g	11	1.1	1.9	216.06	109.98	16.38	0.23
	0.33	c							
chopped,	100.00	g	20	1.1	4.4	29.00	203.00	29.00	0.23
boiled, drained, no salt	144.00	g	29	1.6	6.3	41.76	292.32	41.76	0.33
	1.00	c							
canned, with no salt	100.00	g	19	1.4	2.8	29.00	141.00	21.00	0.30
	144.00	g	27	2.0	4.1	41.76	203.04	30.24	0.43
	1.00	c							
frozen, chopped, boiled, drained, no salt added	100.00	g	29	3.4	5.0	15.00	224.00	34.00	0.42
	164.00	g	48	5.5	8.2	24.60	367.36	55.76	0.69
	1.00	c							

RUTABAGA

	SERVING QUANTITY	SERVING UNIT	CALORIES (kcal)	PROTEIN (g)	TOTAL CARBOHYDRATES (g)	SODIUM (mg)	POTASSIUM (mg)	PHOSPHORUS (mg)	TOTAL FAT (g)
raw, cubes	100.00	g	37	1.1	8.6	12.00	305.00	53.00	0.16
	93.33	g	35	1.0	8.1	11.20	284.67	49.47	0.15
	0.67	c							
boiled, drained, no salt cubed	100.00	g	30	0.9	6.8	5.00	216.00	41.00	0.18
	170.00	g	51	1.6	11.6	8.50	367.20	69.70	0.31
	1.00	c							
boiled, drained, mashed	100.00	g	30	0.9	6.8	5.00	216.00	41.00	0.18
	160.80	g	48	1.5	11.0	8.04	347.33	65.93	0.29
	0.67	c							

PARSNIPS

	SERVING QUANTITY	SERVING UNIT	CALORIES (kcal)	PROTEIN (g)	TOTAL CARBOHYDRATES (g)	SODIUM (mg)	POTASSIUM (mg)	PHOSPHORUS (mg)	TOTAL FAT (g)
raw, sliced	100.00	g	75	1.2	18.0	10.00	375.00	71.00	0.30
	88.67	g	67	1.1	16.0	8.87	332.50	62.95	0.27
	0.67	c							
boiled, drained, sliced, no salt	100.00	g	71	1.3	17.0	10.00	367.00	69.00	0.30
	78.00	g	55	1.0	13.3	7.80	286.26	53.82	0.23
	0.50	c							

WATER CHESTNUTS	SERVING QUANTITY	SERVING UNIT	CALORIES (kcal)	PROTEIN (g)	TOTAL CARBOHYDRATES (g)	SODIUM (mg)	POTASSIUM (mg)	PHOSPHORUS (mg)	TOTAL FAT (g)
fresh, raw,	100.00	g	97	1.4	23.9	14.00	584.00	63.00	0.10
Chinese (Matai) slices	62.00	g	60	0.9	14.8	8.68	362.08	39.06	0.06
	0.50	c							
canned with	100.00	g	50	0.9	12.3	8.00	118.00	19.00	0.06
liquid Chinese (Matai)	70.00	g	35	0.6	8.6	5.60	82.60	13.30	0.04
	0.50	c							
WATERCRESS									
raw, chopped	100.00	g	11	2.3	1.3	41.00	330.00	60.00	0.10
	34.00	g	4	0.8	0.4	13.94	112.20	20.40	0.03
	1.00	c							
YAM									
raw, in cubes	100.00	g	118	1.5	28.0	9.00	816.00	55.00	0.17
	112.50	g	133	1.7	31.4	10.13	918.00	61.88	0.19
	0.75	c							
baked or	100.00	g	116	1.5	27.5	8.00	670.00	49.00	0.14
broiled, drained, no salt cubed	68.00	g	79	1.0	18.7	5.44	455.60	33.32	0.10
	0.50	c							
Hawaiin	100.00	g	67	1.3	16.3	13.00	418.00	34.00	0.10
Mountain, raw cubed	68.00	g	46	0.9	11.1	8.84	284.24	23.12	0.07
	0.50	c							
Hawaiian	100.00	g	82	1.7	20.0	12.00	495.00	40.00	0.08
Mountain, steamed cubed	145.00	g	119	2.5	29.0	17.40	717.75	58.00	0.12
	1.00	c							
MIXED VEGETABLES									
frozen	100.00	g	72	3.3	13.5	47.00	212.00	59.00	0.52
	72.00	g	52	2.4	9.7	33.84	152.64	42.48	0.37
	0.50	c							
frozen, boiled,	100.00	g	65	2.9	13.1	35.00	169.00	51.00	0.15
drained, no salt added	91.00	g	59	2.6	11.9	31.85	153.79	46.41	0.14
	0.50	c							
canned, drained	100.00	g	49	2.6	9.3	214.00	291.00	42.00	0.25
	163.00	g	80	4.2	15.1	348.82	474.33	68.46	0.41
	1.00	c							
BRUSSEL SPROUTS									
raw	100.00	g	43	33.4	9.0	25.00	389.00	69.00	0.30
	88.00	g	38	3.0	7.9	22.00	342.00	60.70	0.26
	1.00	c							

SWISS CHARD	SERVING QUANTITY	SERVING UNIT	CALORIES (kcal)	PROTEIN (g)	TOTAL CARBOHYDRATES (g)	SODIUM (mg)	POTASSIUM (mg)	PHOSPHORUS (mg)	TOTAL FAT (g)
raw	100.00	g	19	1.8	3.7	213.00	379.00	46.00	0.20
	36.00	g	7	0.7	1.4	76.68	136.44	16.56	0.07
	1.00	c							
boiled, drained, no salt	100.00	g	20	1.9	4.1	179.00	549.00	33.00	0.08
	175.00	g	35	3.3	7.2	313.25	960.75	57.75	0.14
	1.00	c							
SPINACH									
raw, chopped	100.00	g	23	2.9	3.6	79.00	558.00	49.00	0.39
	90.00	g	21	2.6	3.3	71.10	502.20	44.10	0.35
	3.00	c							
frozen	100.00	g	29	3.6	4.2	74.00	346.00	49.00	0.57
	78.00	g	23	2.8	3.3	57.72	269.88	38.22	0.44
	0.50	c							
chopped, boiled, drained, no salt	100.00	g	23	3.0	3.8	70.00	466.00	56.00	0.26
	90.00	g	21	2.7	3.4	63.00	419.40	50.40	0.23
	0.50	c							
mustard (Tendergreens)	100.00	g	22	2.2	3.9	21.00	449.00	28.00	0.30
	150.00	g	33	3.3	5.9	31.50	673.50	42.00	0.45
	1.00	c							
mustard, boiled, drained, no salt	100.00	g	16	1.7	2.8	14.00	285.00	18.00	0.20
	180.00	g	29	3.1	5.0	25.20	513.00	32.40	0.36
	1.00	c							
TOMATILLOS									
chopped	100.00	g	32	1.0	5.8	1.00	268.00	39.00	1.02
	132.00	g	42	1.3	7.7	1.32	353.76	51.48	1.35
	1.00	c							
TURNIPS									
raw	100.00	g	28	0.9	6.4	67.00	191.00	27.00	0.10
	130.00	g	34	1.1	7.8	81.74	233.02	32.94	0.12
	1.00	c							
frozen	100.00	g	16	1.0	2.9	25.00	137.00	20.00	0.16
	85.05	g	14	0.9	2.5	21.26	116.52	17.01	0.14
	3.00	oz							
cubed, boiled, drained, no salt	100.00	g	22	0.7	5.1	16.00	177.00	40.56	0.08
	156.00	g	34	1.1	7.9	24.96	276.12	26.00	0.12
	1.00	c							
frozen, boiled, drained, no salt	100.00	g	23	1.5	4.4	36.00	182.00	26.00	0.24
	78.00	g	18	1.2	3.4	28.08	141.96	20.28	0.19
	0.50	c							

KALE

	SERVING QUANTITY	SERVING UNIT	CALORIES (Kcal)	PROTEIN (g)	TOTAL CARBOHYDRATES (g)	SODIUM (mg)	POTASSIUM (mg)	PHOSPHORUS (mg)	TOTAL FAT (g)
raw, chopped	100.00	g	35	2.9	4.4	53.00	348.00	55.00	1.49
	83.75	g	29	2.5	3.7	44.39	291.45	46.06	1.25
	1.25	c							
chopped, boiled, drained, no salt	100.00	g	36	2.9	5.3	16.00	144.00	42.00	1.21
	65.00	g	23	1.9	3.5	10.40	93.60	27.30	0.79
	0.50	c							
scotch, raw, chopped	100.00	g	42	2.8	8.3	70.00	450.00	62.00	0.60
	83.75	g	35	2.4	7.0	58.63	376.88	51.93	0.50
	1.25	c							
scotch, boiled, drained, chopped no salt	100.00	g	28	1.9	5.6	45.00	274.00	38.00	0.41
	86.67	g	24	1.7	4.9	39.00	237.47	32.93	0.36
	0.67	c							
frozen, raw 1 pack=10 oz/ 284g	100.00	g	28	2.7	4.9	15.00	333.00	29.00	0.46
	85.05	g	24	2.3	4.2	12.76	283.21	24.66	0.39
	3.00	oz							
frozen, chopped, boiled, drained, no salt	100.00	g	36	2.9	5.3	16.00	144.00	42.00	1.21
	65.00	g	23	1.9	3.5	10.40	93.60	27.30	0.79
	0.50	c							

MUSTARD GREENS

	SERVING QUANTITY	SERVING UNIT	CALORIES (Kcal)	PROTEIN (g)	TOTAL CARBOHYDRATES (g)	SODIUM (mg)	POTASSIUM (mg)	PHOSPHORUS (mg)	TOTAL FAT (g)
raw, chopped	100.00	g	27	2.9	4.7	20.00	384.00	58.00	0.42
	84.00	g	23	2.4	3.9	16.80	322.56	48.72	0.35
	1.50	c							
boiled, drained, chopped, no salt	100.00	g	26	2.6	4.5	9.00	162.00	42.00	0.47
	70.00	g	18	1.8	3.2	6.30	113.40	29.40	0.33
	0.50	c							
frozen 1 pack=10oz/284g	100.00	g	20	2.5	3.4	29.00	170.00	30.00	0.27
	73.00	g	15	1.8	2.5	21.17	124.10	21.90	0.20
	0.50	c							
frozen, boiled, drained, no salt 1 pack = 10oz/ 212g	100.00	g	19	2.3	3.1	25.00	139.00	24.00	0.25
	75.00	g	14	1.7	2.3	18.75	104.25	18.00	0.19
	0.50	c							

F. Fruits

Hey there!

Do you need to print out this Food List?

You can download a printable version of this chart by scanning the QR code below or copying the link on your computer browser.

https://go.renaltracker.com/printfoodlist

APPLE	SERVING QUANTITY	SERVING UNIT	CALORIES (kcal)	PROTEIN (g)	TOTAL CARBOHYDRATES (g)	SODIUM (mg)	POTASSIUM (mg)	PHOSPHORUS (mg)	TOTAL FAT (g)
Gala, raw, with	100.00	g	57	0.3	13.7	1.00	108.00	11.00	0.12
skin	172.00	g	98	0.4	23.5	1.72	185.76	18.92	0.21
	1.00	pc, med							
fuji, raw, with	100.00	g	63	0.2	15.2	1.00	109.00	13.00	0.18
skin	192.00	g	121	0.4	29.2	1.92	209.28	24.96	0.35
	1.00	pc, med							
golden	100.00	g	57	0.3	13.6	2.00	100.00	10.00	0.15
delicious, with	169.00	g	96	0.5	23.0	3.38	169.00	16.90	0.25
skin									
	1.00	pc, med							
granny smith,	100.00	g	58	0.4	13.6	1.00	120.00	12.00	0.19
w/ skin, raw	167.00	g	97	0.7	22.7	1.67	200.40	20.04	0.32
	1.00	pc, med							
juice, frozen	100.00	g	47	0.1	11.5	7.00	126.00	7.00	0.10
concentrate	239.00	g	112	0.3	27.6	16.73	301.14	16.73	0.24
	8.00	fl oz							
applesauce,	100.00	g	68	0.2	17.5	2.00	75.00	6.00	0.17
sweetened,	123.00	g	84	0.2	21.5	2.46	92.25	7.38	0.21
canned									
	0.50	c							
applesauce,	100.00	g	42	0.2	11.3	2.00	74.00	5.00	0.10
unsweetened,									
canned									
	122.00	g	51	0.2	13.8	2.44	90.28	6.10	0.12
	0.50	c							
BLACK BERRIES									
raw	100.00	g	43	1.4	9.6	1.00	162.00	22.00	0.49
	144.00	g	62	2.0	13.8	1.44	233.28	31.68	0.71
	1.00	c							
frozen,	100.00	g	64	1.2	15.7	1.00	140.00	30.00	0.43
unsweetened									
	151.00	g	97	1.8	23.7	1.51	211.40	45.30	0.65
	1.00	c							
canned, heavy	100.00	g	92	1.3	23.1	3.00	99.00	14.00	0.14
syrup									
	256.00	g	236	3.4	59.1	7.68	253.44	35.84	0.36
	1.00	c							

RASP BERRIES	SERVING QUANTITY	SERVING UNIT	CALORIES (kcal)	PROTEIN (g)	TOTAL CARBOHYDRATES (g)	SODIUM (mg)	POTASSIUM (mg)	PHOSPHORUS (mg)	TOTAL FAT (g)
raw	100.00	g	52	1.2	11.9	1.00	151.00	29.00	0.69
	123.00	g	64	1.5	14.7	1.23	185.73	35.67	0.80
	1.00	c							
frozen, unsweetend	100.00	g	56	1.2	12.6	4.00	184.00	30.00	0.81
	140.00	g	78	1.6	17.6	5.60	257.60	42.00	1.13
	1.00	c							
red, frozen, sweetened, unthawed	100.00	g	103	0.7	26.2	1.00	114.00	17.00	0.16
	125.00	g	129	0.9	32.7	1.25	142.50	21.25	0.20
	0.50	c							
puree, with seeds	100.00	g	55	na	11.5	4.00	195.00	30.00	0.97
juice concentrate	100.00	g	221	3.0	53.2	10.0	1,178.0	100.0	1.34

PEARS

	SERVING QUANTITY	SERVING UNIT	CALORIES (kcal)	PROTEIN (g)	TOTAL CARBOHYDRATES (g)	SODIUM (mg)	POTASSIUM (mg)	PHOSPHORUS (mg)	TOTAL FAT (g)
whole, medium (2.5/lb)	100.00	g	57	0.4	15.2	1.00	116.00	16.00	0.14
	166.00	g	95	0.6	25.3	1.66	192.56	19.92	0.23
	1.00	pc							
halves, canned in water	100.00	g	29	0.2	7.8	2.00	53.00	7.00	0.03
	244.00	g	71	0.5	19.1	4.88	129.32	17.08	0.07
	1.00	c							
Asian	100.00	g	42	0.5	10.7	0.00	121.00	11.00	0.23
	122.00	g	51	0.6	13.0	0.00	147.62	13.42	0.28
	1.00	pc							

CRANBERRY

	SERVING QUANTITY	SERVING UNIT	CALORIES (kcal)	PROTEIN (g)	TOTAL CARBOHYDRATES (g)	SODIUM (mg)	POTASSIUM (mg)	PHOSPHORUS (mg)	TOTAL FAT (g)
fresh, chopped	100.00	g	46	0.5	12.0	2.00	80.00	11.00	0.13
	55.00	g	25	0.3	6.6	1.10	44.00	6.05	0.07
	0.50	c							
dried, sweetened	100.00	g	308	0.2	82.8	5.00	49.00	8.00	1.09
	40.00	g	123	0.1	33.1	2.00	19.60	3.20	0.44
	0.33	c							
juice, unsweetened	100.00	g	46	0.4	12.2	2.00	77.00	13.00	0.13
	253.00	g	116	1.0	30.9	5.06	194.81	32.89	0.33
	1.00	c							
juice, cran cocktail	100.00	g	54	0.0	13.5	2.00	14.00	1.00	0.10
	253.00	g	137	0.0	34.2	5.06	35.42	2.53	0.25
	8.00	fl oz							
sauce, canned, sweetened	100.00	g	159	0.9	40.4	5.00	28.00	4.00	0.15
	69.25	g	110	0.6	28.0	3.46	19.39	2.77	0.10
	0.25	c							

BLUE BERRIES

	SERVING QUANTITY	SERVING UNIT	CALORIES (kcal)	PROTEIN (g)	TOTAL CARBOHYDRATES (g)	SODIUM (mg)	POTASSIUM (mg)	PHOSPHORUS (mg)	TOTAL FAT (g)
fresh	100.00	g	57	0.7	14.5	1.00	77.00	12.00	0.33
	145.00	g	83	1.1	21.0	1.45	111.6	17.40	0.48
	1.00	c							
sweetened,	100.00	g	317	2.5	80.0	3.00	214.0	36.00	2.50
dried	40.00	g	127	1.0	32.0	1.20	85.60	14.40	1.00
	0.25	c							
wild, frozen	100.00	g	57	0.0	13.9	3.00	68.00	13.00	0.16
	140.00	g	80	0.0	19.4	4.20	95.20	18.20	0.22
	1.00	c							
unsweetened,	100.00	g	51	0.4	12.2	1.00	54.00	11.00	0.64
frozen	155.00	g	79	0.7	18.9	1.55	83.70	17.05	0.99
	1.00	c							
canned, light	100.00	g	88	1.0	22.7	3.00	54.00	12.00	0.40
syrup, drained	244.00	g	215	2.5	55.3	7.32	131.7	29.28	0.98
	1.00	c							

STRAWBERRIES

	SERVING QUANTITY	SERVING UNIT	CALORIES (kcal)	PROTEIN (g)	TOTAL CARBOHYDRATES (g)	SODIUM (mg)	POTASSIUM (mg)	PHOSPHORUS (mg)	TOTAL FAT (g)
fresh, whole	100.00	g	32	0.7	7.7	1.00	153.0	24.00	0.30
	144.00	g	46	1.0	11.1	1.44	220.3	34.56	0.43
	1.00	c							
unsweetened,	100.00	g	35	0.4	9.1	2.00	148.0	13.00	0.11
frozen	149.00	g	52	0.6	13.6	2.98	220.5	19.37	
(unthawed)									0.16
	1.00	c							
sweetened,	100.00	g	78	0.5	21.0	1.00	98.00	12.00	0.14
frozen, thawed	127.50	g	99	0.7	26.8	1.28	124.9	15.30	0.18
	0.50	c							
fruit topping	100.00	g	254	0.2	66.3	21.00	51.00	5.00	0.10
	42.00	g	107	0.1	27.9	8.82	21.42	2.10	0.04
	2.00	tbsp							
pastry,	100.00	g	371	5.4	47.8	445.00	83.00	89.00	18.50
127pprox,	71.00	g	263	3.8	33.9	315.95	58.93	63.19	13.14
enriched									
	1.00	pc							
Milkshake	100.00	g	113	3.4	18.9	83.00	182.0	100.0	2.80
(fastfood)	226.40	g	256	7.7	42.8	187.91	412.1	226.4	6.34
	8.00	fl oz							
yogurt 127ppro,	100.00	g	105	8.2	12.3	33.00	129.0	109.0	2.57
low fat									
1 item = 1	150.00	g	158	12.3	18.4	49.50	193.5	163.5	3.86
container									
	1.00	item							

PINE APPLE

	SERVING QUANTITY	SERVING UNIT	CALORIES (kcal)	PROTEIN (g)	TOTAL CARBOHYDRATES (g)	SODIUM (mg)	POTASSIUM (mg)	PHOSPHORUS (mg)	TOTAL FAT (g)
traditional varieties, diced	100.00	g	45	0.6	18.3	1.00	125.00	9.00	0.13
	155.00	g	70	0.9	11.8	1.55	193.75	13.95	0.20
	1.00	c							
sweetened, frozen, chunks	100.00	g	86	0.4	22.2	2.00	100.00	4.00	0.10
	245.00	g	211	1.0	54.4	4.90	245.00	9.80	0.25
	1.00	c							
canned in water crushed, sliced, or chunks	100.00	g	32	0.4	8.3	1.00	127.00	4.00	0.09
	246.00	g	79	1.1	20.4	2.46	312.42	9.84	0.22
	1.00	c							
canned in juice crushed, sliced, or chunks	100.00	g	60	0.4	15.7	1.00	122.00	6.00	0.08
	249.00	g	149	1.1	39.1	2.49	303.78	14.94	0.20
	1.00	c							
extra sweet variety, diced	100.00	g	51	0.5	13.5	1.00	108.00	8.00	0.11
	155.00	g	79	0.8	20.9	1.55	167.40	12.40	0.17
	1.00	c							
juice, unsweetened, canned	100.00	g	53	0.4	12.9	2.00	130.00	8.00	0.12
	250.00	g	133	0.9	32.2	5.00	325.00	20.00	0.30
	8.00	fl oz							
canned in light syrup crushed, sliced, or chunks	100.00	g	52	0.4	13.5	1.00	105.00	7.00	0.12
	126.00	g	66	0.5	17.0	1.26	132.30	8.82	0.15
	0.50	c							
juice, unsweetened, frozen concentrate	100.00	g	179	1.3	44.3	3.00	472.00	28.00	0.10
	288.00	g	387	2.8	95.7	6.48	1,019.5	60.48	0.22
	1.00	c							
juice, 128pprox.128ne d with Vit A, C & E	100.00	g	50	0.4	12.2	3.00	132.00	9.00	0.14
	250.00	g	125	0.9	30.5	7.50	330.00	22.50	0.35
	1.00	c							

128

GRAPE

	SERVING QUANTITY	SERVING UNIT	CALORIES (kcal)	PROTEIN (g)	TOTAL CARBOHYDRATES (g)	SODIUM (mg)	POTASSIUM (mg)	PHOSPHORUS (mg)	TOTAL FAT (g)
red or green, seedless	100.00	g	69	0.7	18.1	2.00	191.00	20.00	0.16
	151.00	g	104	1.1	27.3	3.02	288.41	30.20	0.24
	1.00	c							
juice, unsweetened, plus Vit.C	100.00	g	60	0.4	14.8	5.00	104.00	14.00	0.13
	252.80	g	152	0.9	37.3	12.64	262.90	35.39	0.33
	8.00	fl oz							
fruit mixed/ fruit cocktail, light, drained	100.00	g	55	0.4	14.3	6.00	85.00	13.00	0.08
juice, sweetened, frozen concentrate 6 fl oz can	100.00	g	179	0.7	44.4	7.00	74.00	15.00	0.31
	216.00	g	387	1.4	95.8	15.12	159.84	32.40	0.67
	1.00	can/ item							
seedless, Thompson, canned in water	100.00	g	40	0.5	10.3	6.00	107.00	18.00	0.11
	245.00	g	98	1.2	25.2	14.70	262.15	44.10	0.27
	1.00	c							
jelly 1 packet= 14g (0.5oz)	100.00	g	266	0.2	70.0	30.00	54.00	6.00	0.02
	21.00	g	56	0.0	14.7	6.30	11.34	1.26	0.00
	1	tbsp							

GRAPE-FRUIT	SERVING QUANTITY	SERVING UNIT	CALORIES (kcal)	PROTEIN (g)	TOTAL CARBOHYDRATES (g)	SODIUM (mg)	POTASSIUM (mg)	PHOSPHORUS (mg)	TOTAL FAT (g)
fresh	100.00	g	32	0.6	8.1	0.00	139.0	8.00	0.10
	153.33	g	49	1.0	12.4	0.00	213.1	12.27	0.15
	0.67	c							
white, fresh, small (3.5 diameter)	100.00	g	33	0.7	8.4	0.00	148.0	8.00	0.10
	118.00	g	39	0.8	9.9	0.00	174.6	9.44	0.12
	0.50	pc							
pink or red	100.00	g	42	0.8	10.7	0.00	135.0	18.00	0.14
	153.33	g	64	1.2	16.4	0.00	207.0	27.60	0.21
	0.67	c							
juice, white	100.00	g	39	0.5	9.2	1.00	162.0	15.00	0.10
	247.00	g	96	1.2	22.7	2.47	400.2	37.05	0.25
	8.00	fl oz							
juice, pink	100.00	g	39	0.5	9.2	1.00	162.0	15.00	0.10
	247.00	g	96	1.2	22.7	2.47	400.2	37.05	0.25
	1.00	c							
juice, unsweetened, pink, canned	100.00	g	37	0.6	7.5	2.00	141.0	17.00	0.66
	247.20	g	91	1.4	18.6	4.94	348.6	42.02	1.63
	8.00	fl oz							

ELDERBERRIES

	SERVING QUANTITY	SERVING UNIT	CALORIES	PROTEIN	TOTAL CARBOHYDRATES	SODIUM	POTASSIUM	PHOSPHORUS	TOTAL FAT
	100.00	g	73	7.0	18.4	6.00	280.0	39.00	0.50
fresh	145.00	g	106	1.0	26.7	8.70	406.0	56.55	0.73
	1.00	c							

GOOSEBERRIES

fresh	100.00	g	44	0.9	10.2	1.00	198.0	27.00	0.58
	150.00	g	66	1.3	15.3	1.50	297.0	40.50	0.87
	1.00	c							
canned in light syrup	100.00	g	73	0.7	18.8	2.00	77.00	7.00	0.20
	252.00	g	184	1.6	47.3	5.04	194.1	17.64	0.50
	1.00	c							

KIWI (Chinese gooseberries)

fresh, medium, without skin	100.00	g	61	1.1	14.7	3.00	312.0	34.00	0.52
	76.00	g	46	0.9	11.1	2.28	237.1	25.84	0.40
	1.00	pc							

LOGAN BERRIES

frozen	100.00	g	55	1.5	13.0	1.00	145.0	26.00	0.31
	147.00	g	81	2.2	19.1	1.47	213.2	38.22	0.46
	1.00	c							

CHERRIES

CHERRIES	SERVING QUANTITY	SERVING UNIT	CALORIES (kCal)	PROTEIN (g)	TOTAL CARBOHYDRATES (g)	SODIUM (mg)	POTASSIUM (mg)	PHOSPHORUS (mg)	TOTAL FAT (g)
sweet, without	100.00	g	63	1.1	16.0	0.00	222.0	21.00	0.20
pits	154.00	g	97	1.6	24.7	0.00	341.9	32.34	0.31
	1.00	c							
sour red, without	100.00	g	50	1.0	12.2	3.00	173.0	15.00	0.30
pits	155.00	g	78	1.6	18.9	4.65	268.2	23.25	0.47
	1.00	c							
juice, tart	100.00	g	59	0.3	13.7	4.00	161.0	17.00	0.54
	269.00	g	159	0.8	36.9	10.76	433.1	45.73	1.45
	1.00	c							
Pitanga or	100.00	g	33	0.8	7.5	3.00	103.0	11.00	0.40
Surinam	173.00	g	57	1.4	13.0	5.19	178.2	19.03	0.69
	1.00	c							
tart, dried,	100.00	g	333	1.3	80.5	13.00	376.0	36.00	0.73
sweetened	40.00	g	133	0.5	32.2	5.20	150.4	14.40	0.29
	0.25	c							
maraschino,	100.00	g	165	0.2	42.0	4.00	21.0	3.00	0.21
canned, drained	5.00	g	8	0.0	2.1	0.20	1.05	0.15	0.01
	1.00	pc/ item							
sweet, canned in	100.00	g	54	0.9	13.8	3.00	131.0	22.00	0.02
juice, pitted	250.00	g	135	2.3	34.5	7.50	327.5	55.00	0.05
	1.00	c							
sweet, canned in	100.00	g	46	0.8	11.8	1.00	131.0	15.00	0.13
water	248.00	g	114	1.9	29.2	2.48	324.9	37.20	0.32
	1.00	c							
sweet, frozen,	100.00	g	89	1.2	22.4	1.00	199.0	16.00	0.13
sweetened	259.00	g	231	3.0	57.9	2.59	515.4	41.44	0.34
thawed									
	1.00	c							
pie filling, canned	100.00	g	115	0.4	28.0	18.00	105.0	15.00	0.07
1/8 of 21 oz can	74.00	g	85	0.3	20.7	13.32	77.70	11.10	0.05
	1.00	svg							
pie fillings, low	100.00	g	53	0.8	12.0	12.00	118.0	15.00	0.16
calorie	264.00	g	140	2.2	31.6	31.68	311.5	39.60	0.42
	1.00	c							
sour red, canned	100.00	g	42	0.7	10.5	4.00	115.0	16.00	0.21
in water, drained	168.00	g	71	1.2	17.6	6.72	193.2	26.88	0.35
	1.00	c							
sour red,	100.00	g	46	0.9	11.0	1.00	124.0	16.00	0.44
131pprox.131ned,									
frozen	155.00	g	71	1.4	17.1	1.55	192.2	24.80	0.68
unthawed									
	1.00	c							
sour red, canned	100.00	g	75	0.7	19.3	7.00	95.00	10.00	0.10
in light syrup	126.00	g	95	0.9	24.3	8.82	119.7	12.60	0.13
	0.50	c							

PEACHES

	SERVING QUANTITY	SERVING UNIT	CALORIES (kcal)	PROTEIN (g)	TOTAL CARBOHYDRATES (g)	SODIUM (mg)	POTASSIUM (mg)	PHOSPHORUS (mg)	TOTAL FAT (g)
raw, medium	100.00	g	39	0.9	9.5	0.00	190.0	20.00	0.25
(132pprox. 4/lb)	150.00	g	59	1.4	14.3	0.00	285.0	30.00	0.38
	1.00	pc/ item							
dried	100.00	g	325	4.9	83.2	10.00	1,351	162.0	1.03
	38.67	g	126	1.9	32.2	3.87	522.4	62.64	0.40
	0.33	c							
slices	100.00	g	39	0.9	9.5	0.00	190.0	20.00	0.25
	154.00	g	60	1.4	14.7	0.00	292.6	30.80	0.39
	1.00	c							
nectar, canned	100.00	g	49	0.1	11.6	11.00	30.00	3.00	0.57
	249.00	g	122	0.3	28.9	27.39	74.70	7.47	1.42
	8.00	fl oz							
pie, prepared	100.00	g	224	1.9	33.0	217.00	125.0	22.00	10.00
1/6 of 8-in. pie	117.00	g	262	2.2	38.5	253.89	146.3	25.74	11.70
	1.00	slice							
slices, sweetened, frozen	100.00	g	94	0.6	24.0	6.00	130.0	11.00	0.13
	125.00	g	118	0.8	30.0	7.50	162.5	13.75	0.16
	0.50	c							
halves/ slices, canned in water	100.00	g	24	0.4	6.1	3.00	99.00	10.00	0.06
	122.00	g	29	0.5	7.5	3.66	120.8	12.20	0.07
	0.50	c							
halves/ slices, canned in juice	100.00	g	44	0.6	11.6	4.00	128.0	17.00	0.03
	124.00	g	55	0.8	14.4	4.96	158.7	21.08	0.04
	0.50	c							
canned in extra light syrup	100.00	g	42	0.4	11.1	5.00	74.00	11.00	0.10
	123.50	g	52	0.5	13.7	6.18	91.39	13.59	0.12
	0.50	c							
canned in heavy syrup	100.00	g	75	0.4	20.1	4.00	85.00	9.00	0.10
	242.00	g	182	1.0	48.6	9.68	205.7	21.78	0.24
	1.00	c							
canned in light syrup, drained	100.00	g	61	0.6	15.7	7.00	87.00	10.00	0.15
fruit cocktail, canned light syrup with solids and liquid	100.00	g	55	0.4	14.3	6.00	85.00	13.00	0.08

CANTALOUPE MELON	SERVING QUANTITY	SERVING UNIT	CALORIES (kcal)	PROTEIN (g)	TOTAL CARBOHYDRATES (g)	SODIUM (mg)	POTASSIUM (mg)	PHOSPHORUS (mg)	TOTAL FAT (g)
composite, raw	100.00	g	31	0.7	7.5	8.22	202.4	8.67	0.20
	165.50	g	51	1.1	12.5	13.60	334.9	14.34	0.33
	1.00	c							
honeydew, balls	100.00	g	36	0.5	9.1	18.00	228.0	11.00	0.14
1 slice = 125g	132.75	g	48	0.7	12.1	23.90	302.7	14.60	0.19
	0.75	c							
Navajo	100.00	g	21	0.8	4.1	11.00	140.0	9.00	0.20
	85.05	g	18	0.7	3.5	9.36	119.1	7.65	0.17
	3.00	oz							
melon balls, frozen, unthawed	100.00	g	33	0.8	7.9	31.00	280.0	12.00	0.25
	173.00	g	57	1.5	13.7	53.63	484.4	20.76	0.43
	1.00	c							

BANANA

	SERVING QUANTITY	SERVING UNIT	CALORIES (kcal)	PROTEIN (g)	TOTAL CARBOHYDRATES (g)	SODIUM (mg)	POTASSIUM (mg)	PHOSPHORUS (mg)	TOTAL FAT (g)
medium, 77.8 in long	100.00	g	89	1.1	22.8	1.00	358.0	22.00	0.33
	118.00	g	105	1.3	27.0	1.18	422.5	25.96	0.39
	1.00	pc/ item							
dehydrated, powder	100.00	g	346	3.9	88.3	3.00	1,491	74.00	1.81
	6.20	g	21	0.2	5.5	0.19	92.44	4.59	0.11
	1.00	tbsp							
chips, dried	100.00	g	519	2.3	58.4	6.00	536.0	56.00	14.29
	42.53	g	221	1.0	24.8	2.55	227.9	23.81	33.60
	1.50	oz							
pudding, mix mix to make ½ c 1 package= 88g = 3 ½ oz	100.00	g	366	0.0	93.0	788.00	17.00	5.00	0.40
	22.00	g	81	0.0	20.5	172.36	3.74	1.10	0.09
	1.00	svg							
pudding, ready to eat 1 can = 5 oz	100.00	g	127	2.4	21.2	196.00	110	69.00	3.60
	142.00	g	180	3.4	30.1	278.32	156.2	97.98	5.11
	5.00	oz							

ORANGE	SERVING QUANTITY	SERVING UNIT	CALORIES (kcal)	PROTEIN (g)	TOTAL CARBOHYDRATES (g)	SODIUM (mg)	POTASSIUM (mg)	PHOSPHORUS (mg)	TOTAL FAT (g)
whole, 2-5/8" diameter	100.00	g	47	0.9	11.8	0.00	181.0	14.00	0.12
	131.00	g	62	1.2	15.4	0.00	237.1	18.34	0.16
	1.00	pc/ item							
Valencia (California)	100.00	g	49	1.0	11.9	0.00	179.0	17.00	0.30
	135.00	g	66	1.4	16.1	0.00	241.7	22.95	0.41
	0.75	c							
Navel (California)	100.00	g	49	0.9	12.5	1.00	166.0	28.46	0.15
	123.75	g	61	1.1	15.5	1.24	205.4	23.00	0.19
	0.75	c							
Clementines	100.00	g	47	0.9	12.0	1.00	177.0	21.00	0.15
	74.00	g	35	0.6	8.9	0.74	130.9	15.54	0.11
	1.00	pc/ item							
orange sections	100.00	g	47	0.9	11.8	0.00	181.0	14.00	0.12
	135.00	g	63	1.3	15.9	0.00	244.4	18.90	0.16
	0.75	c							
juice	100.00	g	45	0.7	10.4	1.00	200.0	17.00	0.20
	248.00	g	112	1.7	25.8	2.48	496.0	42.16	0.50
	8.00	fl oz							
Florida, sections 1 fruit = 141g	100.00	g	46	0.7	11.5	0.00	169.0	12.00	0.21
	138.75	g	64	1.0	16.0	0.00	234.5	16.65	0.29
	0.75	c							
soda	100.00	g	48	0.0	12.3	12.00	2.00	1.00	0.00
	248.00	g	119	0.0	30.5	29.76	4.96	2.48	0.00
	8.00	fl oz							
marmalade	100.00	g	246	0.3	66.3	56.00	37.00	4.00	0.00
	20.00	g	49	0.1	13.3	11.20	7.40	0.80	0.00
	1.00	tbsp							
juice, frozen	100.00	g	95	0.5	23.2	8.00	100.0	13.00	0.00
	238.40	g	70	0.4	17.2	5.92	74.00	9.62	0.00
	1.00	c							
orange peel zest	100.00	g	97	1.5	25.0	3.00	212.0	21.00	0.20
	2.00	g	2	0.0	0.5	0.06	4.24	0.42	0.00
	1.00	tsp							
juice, unsweetened, canned	100.00	g	47	0.7	11.0	4.00	184.0	17.00	0.15
	249.00	g	117	1.7	27.4	9.96	458.2	42.33	0.37
	8.00	fl oz							
Mandarin, canned in juice	100.00	g	37	0.6	9.6	5.00	133.0	10.00	
	249.00	g	92	1.5	23.8	12.45	331.2	24.90	
	1.00	c							
juice, light, no pulp	100.00	g	21	0.2	5.4	4.00	188.0	4.00	
	240.00	g	50	0.5	13.0	9.60	451.2	9.60	
	8.00	fl oz							
Mandarin, canned in light syrup	100.00	g	61	0.5	16.2	6.00	78.00	10.00	
	252.00	g	154	1.1	40.8	15.12	196.6	25.20	
	1.00	c							

LEMON	SERVING QUANTITY	SERVING UNIT	CALORIES (kcal)	PROTEIN (g)	TOTAL CARBOHYDRATES (g)	SODIUM (mg)	POTASSIUM (mg)	PHOSPHORUS (mg)	TOTAL FAT (g)
whole, without seeds	100	g	20	1.2	10.7	3.00	145.0	15.00	0.30
	108.00	g	22	1.3	11.6	3.24	156.6	16.20	0.32
	1.00	pc/ item							
peeled, 2-1/8" in diameter)	100.00	g	29	1.1	9.3	2.00	138.0	16.00	0.30
	58.00	g	17	0.6	5.4	1.16	80.04	9.28	0.17
	1.00	pc/ item							
juice, fresh	100.00	g	22	0.4	6.9	1.00	103.0	8.00	0.24
	30.50	g	7	0.1	2.1	0.31	31.42	2.44	0.07
	1.00	fl oz							
peel or zest	100.00	g	47	1.5	16.0	6.00	160.0	12.00	0.30
	2.00	g	1	0.0	0.3	0.12	3.20	0.24	0.01
	1.00	tsp							
pudding mix 1 svg = ½ c	100.00	g	363	0.1	91.8	506.00	5.00	3.00	0.50
1 package = 85g	21.20	g	77	0.0	19.5	107.27	1.06	0.64	0.11
	1.00	svg							
juice, canned	100.00	g	17	0.5	5.6	24.00	109.0	9.00	0.07
	30.50	g	5	0.1	1.7	7.32	33.25	2.75	0.02
	1.00	fl oz							
soda, lemon lime	100.00	g	40	0.1	24.9	9.00	1.00	0.00	0.02
	245.60	g	98	0.1	10.1	22.10	2.46	0.00	0.05
	8.00	fl oz							
juice, unsweetened, frozen	100.00	g	22	0.5	6.5	1.00	89.00	8.00	0.32
	5.08	g	1	0.0	0.3	0.05	4.52	0.41	0.02
	1.00	tsp							
pudding, ready to eat	100.00	g	125	0.1	25.0	140.00	1.00	5.00	3.00
1 can= 5 oz	142.00	g	178	0.1	35.5	198.80	1.42	7.10	4.26
	1.00	can/ item							
tea, black, sweetened, ready to drink	100.00	g	45	0.0	10.8	3.00	14.00	1.00	0.22
	271.00	g	122	0.0	29.3	8.13	37.94	2.71	0.60
	1.00	c							

135

LIME

	SERVING QUANTITY	SERVING UNIT	CALORIES (kcal)	PROTEIN (g)	TOTAL CARBOHYDRATES (g)	SODIUM (mg)	POTASSIUM (mg)	PHOSPHORUS (mg)	TOTAL FAT (g)
whole, 2" in diameter	100.00	g	30	0.7	10.5	2.00	102.0	18.00	0.20
	67.00	g	20	0.5	7.1	1.34	68.34	12.06	0.13
	1.00	pc/ item							
juice, fresh	100.00	g	25	0.4	8.4	2.00	117.0	14.00	0.07
	5.13	g	1	0.0	0.4	0.10	6.01	0.72	0.00
	1.00	tsp							
juice, unsweetened, canned	100.00	g	21	0.3	6.7	16.00	75.00	10.00	0.23
	246.00	g	52	0.6	16.5	39.36	184.5	24.60	0.57
	1.00	c							
frozen ice dessert	100.00	g	128	0.4	32.6	22.00	3.00	1.00	0.00
	99.00	g	127	0.4	32.3	21.78	2.97	0.99	0.00
	0.50	c							

LYCHEE

whole, fresh	100.00	g	66	0.8	16.5	1.00	171.0	31.00	0.44
	142.50	g	94	1.2	23.6	1.43	243.7	44.18	0.63
	0.75	c							
dried	100.00	g	277	3.8	70.7	3.00	1,110	181.00	1.20
	40.00	g	111	1.5	28.3	1.20	444.0	72.40	0.48
	16.00	pcs/ items							

MANGO

whole, fresh	100.00	g	60	0.8	15.0	1.00	168.0	14.00	0.38
	207.00	g	124	1.7	31.0	2.07	347.8	28.98	0.79
	1.00	pc/ item							
dired, sweetened	100.00	g	319	2.5	78.6	162.00	279.0	50.00	1.18
nectar, canned	100.00	g	51	0.1	13.1	5.00	24.00	2.00	0.06
	251.00	g	128	0.3	32.9	12.55	60.24	5.02	0.15
	1.00	c							

136

APRICOT	SERVING QUANTITY	SERVING UNIT	CALORIES (kcal)	PROTEIN (g)	TOTAL CARBOHYDRATES (g)	SODIUM (mg)	POTASSIUM (mg)	PHOSPHORUS (mg)	TOTAL FAT (g)
whole, fresh	100.00	g	48	1.4	11.1	1.00	259.0	23.00	0.39
	140.00	g	67	2.0	15.6	1.40	362.6	32.20	0.55
	4.00	pcs/ items							
jam or preserves	100.00	g	242	0.7	64.4	40.00	77.00	3.00	0.20
1 packet = 0.5 oz = 14g	20.00	g	48	0.1	12.9	8.00	15.40	0.60	0.04
	1.00	tbsp							
nectar, canned	100.00	g	56	0.2	13.6	8.00	67.00	5.00	0.45
	251.00	g	141	0.4	34.2	20.08	168.2	12.55	1.13
	8.00	fl oz							
sweetened, frozen	100.00	g	98	0.7	25.1	4.00	229.0	19.00	0.10
	242.00	g	237	1.7	60.7	9.68	554.2	45.98	0.24
	1.00	c							
dehydrated, sulfured	100.00	g	320	4.9	82.9	13.00	1,850	157.00	0.62
	30.00	g	96	1.5	24.9	3.90	555.0	47.10	0.19
	0.25	c							
dried, halves, sulfured	100.00	g	241	3.4	62.6	10.00	1,162	71.00	0.51
	43.33	g	104	1.5	27.1	4.33	503.5	30.77	0.22
	0.33	c							
halves w/ skin, canned in juice	100.00	g	48	0.6	12.3	4.00	165.0	20.00	0.04
	244.00	g	117	1.5	30.1	9.76	402.6	48.80	0.10
	1.00	c							
halves with skin, canned in light syrup	100.00	g	63	0.5	16.5	4.00	138.0	32.89	0.05
	253.00	g	159	1.3	41.7	10.12	349.1	13.00	0.13
	1.00	c							
PLUM									
whole, fresh, sliced	100.00	g	46	0.7	11.4	0.00	157.0	16.00	0.28
	165.00	g	76	1.2	18.8	0.00	259.1	26.40	0.46
	1.00	c							
sauce	100.00	g	184	0.9	42.8	538.00	259.0	22.00	1.04
	19.00	g	35	0.2	8.1	102.22	49.21	4.18	0.20
	1.00	tbsp							
purple, pitted, canned in water	100.00	g	41	0.4	11.0	1.00	126.0	13.00	0.01
	249.00	g	102	1.0	27.5	2.49	313.7	32.37	0.02
	1.00	c							
purple, canned in juice	100.00	g	58	0.5	15.2	1.00	154.0	15.00	0.02
	252.00	g	146	1.3	38.2	2.52	388.1	37.80	0.05
	1.00	c							

	SERVING QUANTITY	SERVING UNIT	CALORIES (kcal)	PROTEIN (g)	TOTAL CARBOHYDRATES (g)	SODIUM (mg)	POTASSIUM (mg)	PHOSPHORUS (mg)	TOTAL FAT (g)
PRUNE									
puree	100.00	g	257	2.1	65.1	23.00	852.00	72.00	0.20
	28.35	g	73	0.6	18.5	6.52	241.54	20.41	0.06
	1.00	oz							
dried	100.00	g	240	2.2	63.9	2.00	732.00	69.00	0.38
	42.50	g	102	0.9	27.2	0.85	311.10	29.33	0.16
	0.25	c							
juice, canned	100.00	g	71	0.6	17.5	4.00	276.00	25.00	0.03
	256.00	g	182	1.6	44.7	10.24	706.56	64.00	0.08
	8.00	fl oz							
dehydrated, stewed	100.00	g	113	1.2	29.7	2.00	353.00	37.00	0.24
	36.40	g	41	0.5	10.8	0.73	128.49	13.47	0.09
	0.13	c							
dehydrated, low moisture	100.00	g	339	3.7	89.1	5.00	1,058	112.00	0.73
	33.00	g	112	1.2	29.4	1.65	349.14	36.96	0.24
	0.25	c							
RHUBARB									
whole, fresh, diced	100.00	g	21	0.9	4.5	4.00	288.00	14.00	0.20
	81.33	g	17	0.7	3.7	3.25	234.24	11.39	0.16
	0.67	c							
diced, frozen	100.00	g	21	0.6	5.1	2.00	108.00	12.00	0.11
	137.00	g	29	0.8	7.0	2.74	147.96	16.44	0.15
	1.00	c							
frozen, cooked with sugar	100.00	g	116	0.4	31.2	1.00	96.00	8.00	0.05
	120.00	g	139	0.5	37.4	1.20	115.20	9.60	0.06
	0.50	c							
POMEGRANATE									
whole, fresh, 4" in diameter	100.00	g	83	1.7	18.7	3.00	236.00	36.00	1.17
	282.00	g	234	4.7	52.7	8.46	665.52	101.52	3.30
	1.00	pc/ item							
juice, bottled	100.00	g	54	0.2	13.1	9.00	214.00	11.00	0.29
	251.20	g	136	0.4	33.0	22.61	537.57	27.63	0.73
	8.00	fl oz							

PLANTAIN	SERVING QUANTITY	SERVING UNIT	CALORIES (kcal)	PROTEIN (g)	TOTAL CARBOHYDRATES (g)	SODIUM (mg)	POTASSIUM (mg)	PHOSPHORUS (mg)	TOTAL FAT (g)
ripe, raw, fresh	100.00	g	122	1.3	31.9	4.00	487.00	32.00	0.35
	180.00	g	220	2.3	57.4	7.20	877.00	57.60	0.63
	1.00	pc/ item							
green, raw,	100.00	g	152	1.3	36.7	2.00	431.00	31.00	0.07
fresh	267.00	g	406	3.3	97.9	5.34	1,150.0	82.80	0.19
	1.00	pc/item							
green, boiled	100.00	g	121	1.1	29.2	2.00	289.00	24.00	0.08
	137.00	g	166	1.5	39.9	2.74	396.00	32.90	0.11
	1.00	c							
green, fried	100.00	g	309	1.5	49.2	2.00	482.00	44.00	11.81
	118.00	g	365	1.8	58.0	2.36	569.00	51.90	13.90
	1.00	c							
yellow, raw,	100.00	g	122	1.3	31.9	4.00	487.00	32.00	0.35
fresh	270.00	g	329	3.5	86.1	10.8	1,310.0	86.40	0.95
	1.00	pc/ item							
yellow, baked	100.00	g	155	1.5	41.4	2.00	477.00	37.00	0.16
	139.00	g	215	2.1	57.5	2.78	663.00	51.40	0.22
	1.00	c							
chips	100.00	g	531	2.3	63.8	202	786.00	78.00	29.59
	28.35	g	151	0.6	18.1	57.3	223.00	22.10	8.39
	1.00	oz							
AVOCADO									
fresh, raw	100.00	g	160	2.0	8.5	7.00	485.00	52.00	14.66
mashed/ pureed	230.00	g	368	4.6	19.6	16.1	1,120.0	120.0	33.70
	1.00	c							
oil	100.00	g	884	0.0	0.0	0.00	0.00	0.00	100.00
	14.00	g	124	0.0	0.0	0.00	0.00	0.00	14.00
	1.00	tbsp							
dressing	100.00	g	427	1.9	7.4	867	58.00	31.00	43.33
	15.30	g	65	0.3	1.1	133.	8.87	4.74	6.63
	1.00	tbsp							
California, raw/fresh no seed and skin	100.00	g	167	2.0	8.6	8.00	507.00	54.00	15.41
	136.00	g	227	2.7	11.8	10.9	690.00	73.40	21.00
	1.00	pc/ item							
Florida, fresh/ raw no seed and skin	100.00	g	120	2.2	7.8	2.00	351.00	40.00	10.06
	304.00	g	365	6.8	23.8	6.08	1,070.0	122.0	30.60
	1.00	pc/ item							
Guacamole	100.00	g	155	2.0	8.5	344	472.00	51.00	14.18
	15.00	G	23	0.3	1.3	51.6	70.80	7.65	2.13
	1.00	tbsp							

PAPAYA	SERVING QUANTITY	SERVING UNIT	CALORIES (kcal)	PROTEIN (g)	TOTAL CARBOHYDRATES (g)	SODIUM (mg)	POTASSIUM (mg)	PHOSPHORUS (mg)	TOTAL FAT (g)
whole, fresh,	100.00	g	43	0.5	10.8	8.00	182.00	10.00	0.26
cubes	140.00	g	60	0.7	15.2	11.20	254.80	14.00	0.36
	1.00	c							
nectar, canned	100.00	g	57	0.2	14.5	5.00	31.00	0.00	0.15
	250.00	g	143	0.4	36.3	12.50	77.50	0.00	0.38
	8.00	fl oz							
canned with	100.00	g	206	0.1	55.8	9.00	67.00	6.00	0.55
heavy syrup,	39.00	g	80	0.1	21.8	3.51	26.13	2.34	0.21
drained									
	1.00	pc/ chunk							

NECTARINE

	SERVING QUANTITY	SERVING UNIT	CALORIES (kcal)	PROTEIN (g)	TOTAL CARBOHYDRATES (g)	SODIUM (mg)	POTASSIUM (mg)	PHOSPHORUS (mg)	TOTAL FAT (g)
whole, fresh,	100.00	g	44	1.1	10.6	0.00	201.00	26.00	0.32
slices									
	138.00	g	61	1.5	14.7	0.00	277.38	35.88	0.44
	1.00	c							

PERSIMMON

	SERVING QUANTITY	SERVING UNIT	CALORIES (kcal)	PROTEIN (g)	TOTAL CARBOHYDRATES (g)	SODIUM (mg)	POTASSIUM (mg)	PHOSPHORUS (mg)	TOTAL FAT (g)
whole, fresh	100.00	g	127	0.8	33.5	1.00	310.00	26.00	0.40
	25.00	g	32	0.2	8.4	0.25	77.50	6.50	0.10
	1.00	pc/ item							
Japanese, fresh,	100.00	g	70	0.6	18.6	1.00	161.00	17.00	0.19
2-1/2" in	168.00	g	118	1.0	31.2	1.68	270.48	28.56	0.32
diameter									
	1.00	pc/item							
Japanese, dried	100.00	g	274	1.4	73.4	2.00	802.00	81.00	0.59
	34.00	g	93	0.5	25.0	0.68	272.68	27.54	0.20
	1.00	pc/ item							

PURPLE PASSION FRUIT/
GRANADILLA

	SERVING QUANTITY	SERVING UNIT	CALORIES (kcal)	PROTEIN (g)	TOTAL CARBOHYDRATES (g)	SODIUM (mg)	POTASSIUM (mg)	PHOSPHORUS (mg)	TOTAL FAT (g)
whole, fresh –	100.00	g	97	2.2	23.4	28.00	348.00	68.00	0.70
no refuse	18.00	g	18	0.4	4.2	5.04	62.60	12.20	0.13
	1.00	pc/ fruit							
nectar, no ice	100.00	g	67	1.2	17.4	4.00	112.00	5.00	0.06
	31.00	g	21	0.1	5.4	1.24	34.70	1.55	0.02
	1.00	fl oz							
juice, purple	100.00	g	51	0.4	13.6	6.00	278.00	13.00	0.05
passion fruit	30.90	g	16	0.1	4.2	1.85	85.90	4.02	0.02
	1.00	fl oz							
juice, yellow	100.00	g	60	0.7	14.5	6.00	278.00	25.00	0.18
passion fruit	30.90	g	19	0.2	4.5	1.85	85.90	7.72	0.06
	1.00	fl oz							

WATER MELON	SERVING QUANTITY	SERVING UNIT	CALORIES (kcal)	PROTEIN (g)	TOTAL CARBOHYDRATES (g)	SODIUM (mg)	POTASSIUM (mg)	PHOSPHORUS (mg)	TOTAL FAT (g)
raw, balls	100.00	g	30	0.6	7.6	1.00	112.00	11.00	0.15
	154.00	g	46	0.9	11.6	1.54	172.00	16.00	0.23
	1.00	c							
juice, 100%, no	100.00	g	30	0.6	7.6	1.00	112.00	11.00	0.15
ice	30.00	g	9	0.2	2.3	0.30	33.60	3.30	0.05
	1.00	fl oz							
seeds, kernels,	100.00	g	557	28.3	15.3	99.00	648.00	755.0	47.37
dried	28.35	g	158	8.0	4.3	28.10	184.00	214.0	13.4C
	1.00	oz							
FIG									
raw	100.00	g	74	0.8	19.2	1.00	232.00	14.00	0.30
	50.00	g	37	0.4	9.6	0.50	116.00	7.00	0.15
	1.00	pc/ item							
dried	100.00	g	249	3.3	63.9	10.00	680.00	67.00	0.92
	8.00	g	20	0.3	5.1	0.80	54.40	5.36	0.07
	1.00	pc							
canned	100.00	g	75	0.6	19.4	1.00	157.00	10.00	0.24
	250.00	g	188	1.4	48.4	2.50	392.00	25.00	0.60
	1.00	c							
dried, stewed	100.00	g	107	1.4	27.6	4.00	294.00	29.00	0.40
	259.00	g	277	3.7	71.4	10.40	761.00	75.10	1.04
	1.00	c							
canned, water pack, solids/liquids	100.00	g	53	0.4	14.0	1.00	103.00	10.00	0.10
	248.00	g	131	1.0	34.7	2.48	255.00	24.80	0.25
	1.00	c							
canned, light syrup pack, solids/liquids	100.00	g	69	0.4	18.0	1.00	102.00	10.00	0.10
	252.00	g	174	1.0	45.2	2.52	257.00	25.20	0.25
	1.00	c							
GUAVA									
raw	100.00	g	68	2.6	14.3	2.00	417.00	40.00	0.95
	55.00	g	37	1.4	7.9	1.10	229.00	22.00	0.52
	1.00	pc/ item							
nectar	100.00	g	48	0.3	13.3	6.00	33.00	3.00	0.07
no ice	31.00	g	15	0.1	4.1	1.86	10.20	0.93	0.02
	1.00	fl oz							
paste	100.00	g	280	0.1	77.6	2.00	69.00	3.00	0.27
	20.00	g	56	0.0	14.5	0.40	13.80	0.60	0.05
	1.00	tbsp							

	SERVING QUANTITY	SERVING UNIT	CALORIES (kcal)	PROTEIN (g)	TOTAL CARBOHYDRATES (g)	SODIUM (mg)	POTASSIUM (mg)	PHOSPHORUS (mg)	TOTAL FAT (g)
DATES									
whole, dried	100.00	g	282	2.5	75.0	2.00	656.0	62.00	0.39
	8.00	g	23	0.2	6.0	0.16	52.50	4.96	0.03
	1.00	pc/ item							
Medjool,	100.00	g	277	1.8	75.0	1.00	696.0	62.00	0.15
pitted	24.00	g	67	0.4	18.0	0.24	167.0	14.90	0.04
	1.00	pc/item							
candy	100.00	g	379	4.2	58.1	22.00	540.0	117.0	18.04
	28.35	g	107	1.2	16.5	6.24	153.0	33.20	5.11
	1.00	oz							
POMELO									
whole, fresh	100.00	g	38	0.8	9.6	1.00	216.0	17.00	0.04
section	190.00	g	72	1.4	18.3	1.90	410.0	32.30	0.08
	1.00	c							
MANGOSTEEN									
canned, syrup pack	100.00	g	73	0.4	17.9	7.00	48.00	8.00	0.58
drained	196.00	g	143	0.8	35.1	13.70	94.10	15.70	1.14
	1.00	c							
JACKFRUIT									
raw, fresh	100.00	g	95	1.7	23.3	2.00	448.0	21.00	0.64
slices	165.00	g	157	2.8	38.4	3.30	739.0	34.60	1.06
	1.00	c							
canned, syrup pack	100.00	g	92	0.4	23.9	11.00	96.00	6.00	0.14
drained	178.00	g	164	0.6	42.6	19.60	171.0	10.70	0.25
	1.00	c							
DURIAN									
raw or frozen	100.00	g	147	1.5	27.1	2.00	436.0	39.00	5.33
chopped or diced	243.00	g	357	3.6	65.8	4.86	1,060	94.80	13.00
	1.00	c							
SOURSOP									
raw, pulp	100.00	g	66	1.0	16.8	14.00	278.0	27.00	0.30
	225.00	g	148	2.3	37.9	31.50	626.0	60.80	0.68
	1.00	c							
nectar	100.00	g	59	0.1	14.9	8.00	25.00	2.00	0.17
no ice, pure	31.00	g	18	0.0	4.6	2.48	7.75	0.62	0.05
	1.00	fl oz							

	SERVING QUANTITY	SERVING UNIT	CALORIES (kcal)	PROTEIN (g)	TOTAL CARBOHYDRATES (g)	SODIUM (mg)	POTASSIUM (mg)	PHOSPHORUS (mg)	TOTAL FAT (g)
TAMARIND									
fresh, raw	100.00	g	239	2.8	62.5	28.00	628	113	0.60
	2.00	g	5	0.1	1.3	0.56	12.60	2.26	0.01
	1.00	pc/item							
candy	100.00	g	331	0.0	92.0	1,643	309.0	56.00	0.00
	22.00	g	73	0.0	20.2	361.00	68.00	12.30	0.00
	1.00	tbsp							
dried	100.00	g	254	2.5	66.2	25.00	565	102	0.57
	160.00	g	406	4.0	106	40.00	904	163	0.91
	1.00	c							
SAPODILLA									
fresh/raw	100.00	g	83	0.4	20.0	12.00	193	12.00	1.10
	170.00	g	141	0.8	33.9	20.40	328	20.40	1.87
	1.00	pc/ item							
SUGARAPPLE **(Sweetsop)**									
fresh, raw	100.00	g	94	2.1	23.6	9.00	247	32.00	0.29
(2-7/8" in diameter)	155.00	g	146	3.2	36.6	14.00	383	49.60	0.45
	1.00	pc/ item							
STARFRUIT									
fresh/ raw	100.00	g	31	1.0	6.7	2.00	133	12.00	0.33
	90.00	g	28	0.9	6.1	1.80	120.0	10.80	0.30
	1.00	pc/ item							

G. Herbs and Spices

Hey there!

Do you need to print out this Food List?

You can download a printable version of this chart by scanning the QR code below or copying the link on your computer browser.

https://go.renaltracker.com/printfoodlist

	SERVING QUANTITY	SERVING UNIT	CALORIES (kcal)	PROTEIN (g)	TOTAL CARBOHYDRATES (g)	SODIUM (mg)	POTASSIUM (mg)	PHOSPHORUS (mg)	TOTAL FAT (g)
SAGE									
ground	100	g	315	10.6	60.7	11	1070	91	12.8
1 Tbsp	2	g	6.3	0.21	1.21	0.22	21.4	1.82	0.256
CINNAMON									
ground	100	g	247	3.99	80.6	10	431	64	1.24
1 Tbsp	7.8	g	19.3	0.31	6.29	0.78	33.6	4.99	0.097
CUMIN									
seed	100	g	375	17.8	44.2	168	1790	499	22.3
1 Tbsp Whole	6	g	22.5	1.07	2.65	10.1	107	29.9	1.34
NUTMEG									
ground	100	g	525	5.84	49.3	16	350	213	36.3
1 tsp	7	g	36.8	0.41	3.45	1.12	24.5	14.9	2.54
CLOVES									
ground	100	g	274	5.97	65.5	277	1020	104	13
1tsp	6.5	g	17.8	0.39	4.26	18	66.3	6.76	0.845
PARSLEY									
fresh	100	g	36	2.97	6.33	56	554	58	0.79
dried	100	g	292	26.6	50.6	452	2680	436	5.48
CORIANDER									
seed	100	g	298	12.4	55	35	1270	409	17.8
leaves, raw	100	g	23	2.13	3.67	46	521	48	0.52
THYME									
fresh	100	g	101	5.56	24.4	9	609	106	1.68
dried	100	g	276	9.11	63.9	55	814	201	7.43
LEMON GRASS									
citronella, raw	100	g	99	1.82	25.3	6	723	101	0.49

	SERVING QUANTITY	SERVING UNIT	CALORIES (kcal)	PROTEIN (g)	TOTAL CARBOHYDRATES (g)	SODIUM (mg)	POTASSIUM (mg)	PHOSPHORUS (mg)	TOTAL FAT (g)
ONION									
red, raw	100	g	44	0.94	9.93	1	197	41	0.1
1 onion	197	g	86.7	1.85	19.6	1.97	388	80.8	0.197
white, raw	100	g	36	0.89	7.68	2	141	29	0.13
yellow, raw	100	g	38	0.83	8.61	1	182	34	0.05
1 onion	143	g	54.3	1.19	12.3	1.43	260	48.6	0.071
GARLIC									
raw	100	g	149	6.36	33.1	17	401	153	0.5
3 cloves	9	g	13.4	0.572	2.98	1.53	36.1	13.8	0.045
GINGER									
raw	100	g	80	1.82	17.8	13	415	34	0.75
SPRING ONIONS									
raw	100	g	32	1.83	7.34	16	276	37	0.19
1 large	25	g	8	0.458	1.84	4	69	9.25	0.048
CHIVES									
raw	100	g	30	3.27	4.35	3	296	58	0.73
BASIL									
fresh	100	g	23	3.15	2.65	4	295	56	0.64
dried	100	g	233	23	47.8	76	2630	274	4.07
OREGANO									
dried	100	g	265	9	68.9	25	1260	148	4.28
ROSEMARY									
fresh	100	g	131	3.31	20.7	26	668	66	5.86
dried	100	g	331	4.88	64.1	50	995	70	15.2
MARJORAM									
dried	100	g	271	12.7	60.6	77	1520	306	7.04

	SERVING QUANTITY	SERVING UNIT	CALORIES (kcal)	PROTEIN (g)	TOTAL CARBOHYDRATES (g)	SODIUM (mg)	POTASSIUM (mg)	PHOSPHORUS (mg)	TOTAL FAT (g)
FENNEL									
Bulb, raw	100	g	31	1.24	7.3	52	414	50	0.2
seed	100	g	345	15.8	52.3	88	1690	487	14.9
1 Tbsp	5.8	g	20	0.92	3.03	5.1	98	28	0.864
DILL									
weed, fresh	100	g	43	3.46	7.02	61	738	66	1.12
weed, dried	100	g	253	20	55.8	208	3310	543	4.36
1 Tbsp	3.1	g	7.8	0.62	1.73	6.45	103	16.8	0.135
ANISE									
seed	100	g	337	17.6	50	16	1440	440	15.9
1 Tbsp	6.7	g	22.6	1.18	3.35	1.07	96.5	29.5	1.06
CARDAMOM									
spices	100	g	311	10.8	68.5	18	1120	229	6.7
1 Tbsp	5.8	g	18	0.63	3.97	1.04	65	10.3	0.389
CAYENNE									
pepper, red or cayenne	100	g	318	12	56.6	30	2010	293	17.3
1 tbsp	5.3	g	16.9	0.64	3	1.59	107	15.5	0.917
CURRY POWDER									
	100	g	325	14.3	55.8	52	1170	367	14
1 tbsp	6.3	g	20.5	0.90	3.52	3.28	73.7	23.1	0.882
PAPRIKA									
ground	100	g	282	14.1	54	68	2280	314	12.9
1 tbsp	6.8	g	19.2	0.96	3.67	4.62	155	21.4	0.877
CELERY									
celery, raw	100	g	14	0.69	2.97	80	260	24	0.17

147

	SERVING QUANTITY	SERVING UNIT	CALORIES (kcal)	PROTEIN (g)	TOTAL CARBOHYDRATES (g)	SODIUM (mg)	POTASSIUM (mg)	PHOSPHORUS (mg)	TOTAL FAT (g)
SAFFRON									
	100	g	310	11.4	65.4	148	1720	252	5.85
1 tbsp	2.1	g	6.51	0.24	1.37	3.11	36.1	5.29	0.123
PEPPER, BLACK									
ground	100	g	251	10.4	64	20	1330	158	3.26
1 tbsp	6.9	g	17.3	0.72	4.42	1.38	91.8	10.9	0.225
PEPPER, WHITE									
ground	100	g	296	10.4	68.6	5	73	176	2.12
1 tbsp	7.1	g	21	0.74	4.87	0.355	5.18	12.5	0.151
TARRAGON									
dried	100	g	295	22.8	50.2	62	3020	313	7.24
1 Tbsp, leaves	1.8	g	5.31	0.41	0.904	1.12	54.4	5.63	0.13
1 Tbsp, ground	4.8	g	14.2	1.09	2.41	2.98	145	15	0.348
HORSERADISH									
	100	g	48	1.18	11.3	420	246	31	0.69
1 tbsp	15	g	7.2	0.18	1.7	63	36.9	4.65	0.103

H. Carbohydrates

(Grains, Breads, Pasta/Noodles, Cereals)

Hey there!

Do you need to print out this Food List?

You can download a printable version of this chart by scanning the QR code below or copying the link on your computer browser.

https://go.renaltracker.com/printfoodlist

RICE	SERVING QUANTITY	SERVING UNIT	CALORIES (kcal)	PROTEIN (g)	TOTAL CARBOHYDRATES (g)	SODIUM (mg)	POTASSIUM (mg)	PHOSPHORUS (mg)	TOTAL FAT (g)
white, unenriched	100.00	g	359	6.9	79.8	5.00	75.00	94.00	1.30
white, cooked, glutinous	100.00	g	96	2.0	21.0	5.00	20.00	33.00	0.27
	174.00	g	167	3.5	36.5	6.60	26.40	43.60	0.36
	1.00	c							
white, long-grain, parboiled enriched, cooked	100.00	g	123	2.9	26.1	0.00	29.00	37.00	0.21
	158.00	g	194	4.6	41.2	0.00	53.90	68.80	0.39
	1.00	c							
flour, white, unenriched	100.00	g	359	6.9	79.8	0.00	26.00	33.00	0.19
						0.00	53.30	67.60	0.39
white, steamed, Chinese restaurant	100.00	g	151	3.2	33.9				
cup, loosely packed	132.00	g	199	4.2	44.7	1.00	265.0	319.0	3.85
	1.00	c							
white, medium-grain, cooked unenriched	100.00	g	130	2.4	28.6	201.00	86.00	102.00	0.96
	186.00	g	242	4.4	53.2	394.00	169.0	200.0	1.88
	1.00	c							
white, short-grain, cooked unenriched	100.00	g	130	2.4	28.7	3.00	101.0	82.00	0.34
	205.00	g	266	4.8	58.8	4.92	166.0	134.0	0.56
	1.00	c							
flour, brown	100.00	g	365	7.2	75.5	7.00	427.0	433.0	1.08
						11.20	683.0	693.0	1.73
brown, cooked, no salt, no fat	100.00	g	122	2.7	25.5				
	196.00	g	239	5.4	49.9	5.00	75.00	94.00	1.30
	1.00	c							
wild, cooked	100.00	g	101	4.0	21.3	5.00	20.00	33.00	0.27
	164.00	g	166	6.5	35.0	6.60	26.40	43.60	0.36
	1.00	c							
wild, raw	100.00	g	357	14.7	74.9	0.00	29.00	37.00	0.21
	160.00	g	571	23.6	120.0	0.00	53.90	68.80	0.39
	1.00	c							

OATS	SERVING QUANTITY	SERVING UNIT	CALORIES (kcal)	PROTEIN (g)	TOTAL CARBOHYDRATES (g)	SODIUM (mg)	POTASSIUM (mg)	PHOSPHORUS (mg)	TOTAL FAT (g)
raw	100.00	g	379	12.2	67.7	6.00	362.0	410.0	6.52
	81.00	g	307	10.7	54.8	4.86	293.0	332.0	5.28
	1.00	c							
cereal, oat,	100.00	g	372	12.4	73.2	497.00	633.0	357.0	6.60
	33.00	g	123	4.1	24.2	164.00	209.0	118.0	2.18
	1.00	c							
steel cut	100.00	g	378	13.3	66.7	0.00	356.0	na	6.67
Brand:	45.00	g	170	6.0	30.0	0.00	160.0	na	3.00
ARROWHEAD									
MILLS									
	1.00	svg							
rolled	100.00	g	350	12.5	67.5	0.00	350.0	na	6.25
Brand:	40.00	g	140	5.0	27.0	0.00	140.0	na	2.50
MILLVILLE by									
Aldi									
	1.00	svg							
bran, cooked	100.00	g	40	3.2	11.4	1.00	92.00	119.0	0.86
	219.00	g	88	7.0	25.1	2.19	201.0	261.0	1.88
	1.00	c							
bran, uncooked	100.00	g	246	17.3	66.2	4.00	566.0	734.0	7.03
(raw)									
	94.00	g	231	16.3	62.2	3.76	532.0	690.0	6.61
	1.00	c							
flour, partially	100.00	g	404	14.7	65.7	19.00	371.0	452.0	9.12
debranned									
	104.00	g	420	15.2	68.3	19.80	386.0	470.0	9.48
	1.00	c							
regular, rolled,	100.00	g	379	13.2	67.7	6.00	362.0	410.0	6.52
not fortified,									
dry									
	81.00	g	307	10.7	54.8	4.86	293.0	332.0	5.28
	1.00	c							

WHEAT	SERVING QUANTITY	SERVING UNIT	CALORIES (kcal)	PROTEIN (g)	TOTAL CARBOHYDRATES (g)	SODIUM (mg)	POTASSIUM (mg)	PHOSPHORUS (mg)	TOTAL FAT (g)
durum	100.00	g	399	13.7	71.1	2.00	431.0	508.0	2.47
	192.00	g	651	26.3	137	3.84	828.0	975.0	4.74
	1.00	c							
sprouted	100.00	g	198	7.5	42.5	16.00	169.0	200.0	1.27
	108.00	g	214	8.1	45.9	17.30	183.0	216.0	1.37
	1.00	c							
germ	100.00	g	360	23.2	51.8	12.00	892.0	842.0	9.72
	115.00	g	414	26.7	59.6	13.80	1,030	968	11.20
	1.00	c							
bran	100.00	g	216	15.6	64.5	2.00	1,180	1,010	4.25
	58.00	g	125	9.1	37.4	1.16	684.0	586.0	2.46
	1.00	c							
cream of wheat, instant, dry	100.00	g	366	10.6	75.5	571.00	115.0	103.0	1.40
	11.50	g	42	1.2	8.7	65.70	13.20	11.80	0.16
	1.00	tbsp							
flour, whole wheat, unenriched	100.00	g	370	15.1	71.2	3.00	376.0	352.0	2.73
whole grain, soft wheat	100.00	g	332	9.6	74.5	3.00	394.0	323.0	1.95
bread flour, unenriched	100.00	g	361	12.0	72.5	2.00	100.0	97.00	1.66
unsifted	137.00	g	495	16.4	99.4	2.74	137.0	133.0	2.27
	1.00	c							
flour, bread, white, enriched	100.00	g	361	12.0	72.5	2.00	100.0	97.00	1.66
	137.00	g	495	16.4	99.4	2.74	137.0	133.0	2.27
	1.00	c							
fllour, cake, enriched	100.00	g	362	8.2	78.0	2.00	105.0	85.00	0.86
unsifted	137.00	g	496	11.2	107.0	2.74	144.0	116.0	1.18
	1.00	c							

CUOSCUOS

	SERVING QUANTITY	SERVING UNIT	CALORIES (kcal)	PROTEIN (g)	TOTAL CARBOHYDRATES (g)	SODIUM (mg)	POTASSIUM (mg)	PHOSPHORUS (mg)	TOTAL FAT (g)
dry	100.00	g	376	12.8	77.4	10.00	166.0	170.0	0.64
	173.00	g	680	22.1	134	17.30	287.0	294.0	1.11
	1.00	c							
cooked	100.00	g	112	3.8	23.2	5.00	58.00	22.00	0.16
	157.00	g	176	6.0	36.4	7.85	91.10	34.50	0.25
	1.00	c							

BARLEY

	SERVING QUANTITY	SERVING UNIT	CALORIES (kcal)	PROTEIN (g)	TOTAL CARBOHYDRATES (g)	SODIUM (mg)	POTASSIUM (mg)	PHOSPHORUS (mg)	TOTAL FAT (g)
pearled, cooked	100.00	g	123	2.3	28.2	3.00	93.00	54.00	0.44
	157.00	g	193	3.6	44.3	4.71	146.0	84.80	0.69
	1.00	c							
flour or meal	100.00	g	345	10.5	74.5	4.00	309.0	296.0	1.60
	148.00	g	511	15.5	110.	5.92	457.0	438.0	2.37
	1.00	c							

QUINOA

	SERVING QUANTITY	SERVING UNIT	CALORIES (kcal)	PROTEIN (g)	TOTAL CARBOHYDRATES (g)	SODIUM (mg)	POTASSIUM (mg)	PHOSPHORUS (mg)	TOTAL FAT (g)
cooked	100.00	g	120	4.4	21.3	7.00	172.0	152.0	1.92
	185.00	g	222	8.1	39.4	13.00	318.0	281.0	3.55
	1.00	c							
uncooked	100.00	g	368	14.1	64.2	5.00	563.0	457.0	6.07
	170.00	g	626	24.0	109	8.50	957.0	777.0	10.3C
	1.00	c							
pasta from quinoa flour (gluten-free)	100.00	g	152	3.2	31.1	4.00	63.00	91.00	2.07
	132.00	g	201	4.3	41.1	5.28	83.20	120.0	2.73
not packed	1.00	c							

AMARANTH

	SERVING QUANTITY	SERVING UNIT	CALORIES (kcal)	PROTEIN (g)	TOTAL CARBOHYDRATES (g)	SODIUM (mg)	POTASSIUM (mg)	PHOSPHORUS (mg)	TOTAL FAT (g)
Grain	100.00	g	102	3.8	18.7	6.00	135.0	148.0	1.58
cooked	246.00	g	251	9.4	46.0	14.80	332.0	364.0	3.89
	1.00	c							

CEREALS	SERVING QUANTITY	SERVING UNIT	CALORIES (kcal)	PROTEIN (g)	TOTAL CARBOHYDRATES (g)	SODIUM (mg)	POTASSIUM (mg)	PHOSPHORUS (mg)	TOTAL FAT (g)
corn flakes, plain (store brands)	100.00	g	357	7.5	84.1	729.00	168.0	102.0	0.40
	25.00	g	89	1.9	21.0	182.00	42.00	25.50	0.10
	1.00	c							
corn flakes, frosted (store brands)	100.00	g	389	4.3	90.2	451.00	82.00	46.00	0.87
	40.00	g	156	1.7	36.1	180.00	32.80	18.40	0.35
	1.00	c							
crsipy rice	100.00	g	383	6.7	86.2	545.00	106.0	98.00	1.26
	26.00	g	100	1.7	22.4	142.00	27.60	25.50	0.33
	1.00	c							
cocoa puffs (General Mills)	100.00	g	383	5.6	83.7	564.00	272.0	222.0	5.20
	36.00	g	138	2.0	30.1	203.00	97.90	79.90	1.87
	1.00	c							
muesli, with fruits & nuts	100.00	g	335	8.6	74.9	239.00	324.0	225.0	5.40
	85.00	g	302	7.3	63.7	203.00	275.0	191.0	4.59
	1.00	c							
muesli Brand: Safeway	100.00	g	386	8.8	73.7	228.00	474.0	175.0	5.26
	57.00	g	220	5.0	42.0	130.00	270.0	99.80	3.00
	1.00	svg							
granola, homemade, ready-to-eat	100.00	g	489	13.7	53.9	26.00	539.0	431.0	24.30
	122.00	g	597	16.7	65.8	31.70	658.0	526.0	29.60
	1.00	c							
granola bars, plain	100.00	g	471	10.1	64.4	294.00	336.0	277.0	19.80
	28.00	g	132	2.8	18.0	82.30	94.10	77.60	5.54
	1.00	bar/ oz							
granola bars, almond	100.00	g	495	7.7	62.0	256.00	273.0	228.0	25.50
	28.35	g	140	2.2	17.6	72.60	77.40	64.60	7.23
	1.00	oz							

154

PANCAKE	SERVING QUANTITY	SERVING UNIT	CALORIES (kCal)	PROTEIN (g)	TOTAL CARBOHYDRATES (g)	SODIUM (mg)	POTASSIUM (mg)	PHOSPHORUS (mg)	TOTAL FAT (g)
buttermilk	100.00	g	227	6.8	28.7	522.00	145.0	139.0	9.30
(from recipe)	38.00 1- 4" diameter	g pc	86	2.6	10.9	198.00	55.10	52.80	3.53
plain, (prepared from recipe)	100.00	g	227	6.4	28.3	439.00	132.0	159.0	9.70
	38.00 1- 4" diameter	g pc	86	2.4	10.8	167.00	50.20	60.40	3.69
plain, reduced fat	100.00	g	269	5.7	57.3	429.00	97.00	190.0	1.90
	105.00 3.00	g pcs	282	6.0	60.2	450.00	102.0	200.0	2.00
plain, frozen, ready to heat includes buttermilk	100.00	g	233	5.2	37.8	461.00	90.00	215.0	6.83
	40.00 1 (4")	g pc	93	2.1	15.1	184.00	36.00	86.00	2.73
gluten-free, frozen, ready to heat	100.00	g	215	3.3	40.3	331.00	127.0	306.0	4.55
	48.00 1.00	g pc	103	1.6	19.3	159.00	61.00	147.0	2.18
WAFFLE									
plain, prepared from recipe	100.00	g	291	7.9	32.9	511.00	159.0	190.0	14.10
	75.00 1 (7")	g pc	218	5.9	24.7	383.00	119.0	142.0	10.60

BREADS

	SERVING QUANTITY	SERVING UNIT	CALORIES (kcal)	PROTEIN (g)	TOTAL CARBOHYDRATES (g)	SODIUM (mg)	POTASSIUM (mg)	PHOSPHORUS (mg)	TOTAL FAT (g)
whole wheat	100.00	g	252	12.5	42.7	455.0	254	212.0	3.50
	50.00	g	126	6.2	21.4	227.5	127.0	106.0	1.75
	2.00	slices							
white	100.00	g	266	8.9	49.4	490.0	126.0	98.00	490
	50.00	g	133	4.4	24.7	245.0	63.00	49.00	245
	2.00	slices							
french, small (2'x2.5'x1.75')	100.00	g	272	10.8	51.9	602.0	117.0	105.0	2.42
	32.00	g	87	3.4	16.6	192.6	37.44	33.60	0.77
	1.00	slice							
pita, 6.5"	100.00	g	275	9.1	55.7	536.0	120.0	97.00	1.20
	60.00	g	165	5.5	33.4	321.6	72.00	58.20	0.72
	1.00	pc							
sourdough	100.00	g	272	10.8	51.9	602.0	117.0	105.0	2.42
	50.00	g	136	5.4	25.9	301.0	58.50	52.50	1.21
	2.00	slices							
rye	100.00	g	259	8.5	48.3	603.0	166.0	125.0	33.00
	32.00	g	83	2.7	15.5	192.9	53.12	40.00	1.06
	1.00	slice							
bagels, wheat	100.00	g	250	10.2	48.9	439.0	165.0	142.0	1.53
	105.00	g	262	10.7	51.3	461.0	173.0	149.0	1.61
	1.00	reg pc							
biscuits	100.00	g	362	7.5	43.9	930.0	184.0	501.0	18.19
	45.00	g	163	3.4	19.8	418.0	82.80	225.0	8.19
	1.00	pc							
sprouted, wheat	100.00	g	188	13.2	33.9	474.0	198.0	176.0	0.00
	26.00	g	49	3.4	8.8	123.0	51.50	45.80	0.00
	1.00	slice							
cracked, wheat	100.00	g	274	10.7	47.5	473.0	141.0	129.0	4.53
	28.00	g	77	3.0	13.3	132.0	39.50	36.10	1.27
	1.00	reg slice							
tortillas, corn ready-to-bake or fry	100.00	g	218	5.7	44.6	45.00	186.0	314.0	2.85
	24.00	g	52	1.4	10.7	10.80	44.60	75.40	0.68
	1.00	Pc							
tortillas, flour approx. 6" diameter ready-to-bake or fry, refrigerated	100.00	g	306	8.2	49.4	736.0	125.0	206.0	7.99
	30.00	g	92	2.5	14.8	221.0	37.50	61.80	2.40
	1.00	pc							

BREADS	SERVING QUANTITY	SERVING UNIT	CALORIES (kcal)	PROTEIN (g)	TOTAL CARBOHYDRATES (g)	SODIUM (mg)	POTASSIUM (mg)	PHOSPHORUS (mg)	TOTAL FAT (g)
tortilla, whole wheat	100.00	g	310	9.8	45.9	617.00	262.0	346.0	9.76
ready-to-bake or fry	41.00	g	127	4.0	18.8	253.00	107.0	142.0	4.00
	1.00	pc							
ciabatta	100.00	g	259	9.5	48.1	618.00	124.0	95.00	2.73
(yeast bread)	43.00	g	111	4.1	20.7	266.00	53.30	40.80	1.17
italian, grecian, aarmenian thick sllice	1.00	pc							
focaccia, plain	100.00	g	249	8.8	35.8	561.00	114.0	128.0	7.89
(Italian flatbread)	57.00	g	142	5.0	20.4	320.00	65.00	73.00	4.50
	1.00	pc							
Pita, medium	100.00	g	275	9.1	55.7	536.00	120.0	97.00	1.20
	57.00	g	157	5.2	31.7	306.00	68.40	55.30	0.68
	1.00	pc							
Naan, plain	100.00	g	291	9.6	50.4	465.00	125.0	100.0	5.65
	90.00	g	262	8.7	45.4	418.00	112.0	90.00	5.08
	1.00	pc							
Paratha, whole wheat, frozen	100.00	g	326	6.4	45.4	467.00	185.0	188.0	6.70
	79.00	g	258	5.0	35.9	495.00	196.0	199.0	7.10
	1.00	pc							
brioche	100.00	g	418	8.8	35.8	452.00	139.0	120.0	13.20
	77.00	g	322	6.7	27.6	357.00	110.0	94.80	10.40
	1.00	pc							
croissants, plain medium	100.00	g	406	8.2	45.8	440.00	120.0	125.0	26.80
	57.00	g	231	4.7	26.1	339.00	92.40	96.20	20.60
	1.00	pc							
croissants, chocolate	100.00	g	421	7.4	49.4	384.00	118.0	105.0	21.00
	57.00	g	240	4.2	28.2	219.00	67.30	59.80	12.00
	1.00	pc							
croissants, cheese	100.00	g	414	9.2	47.0	361.00	132.0	130.0	20.90
	57.00	g	236	5.2	26.8	206.00	75.22	74.10	11.90
	1.00	pc							
muffins, english, whole grain white	100.00	g	245	7.0	50.2	386.00	130.0	127.0	1.75
	57.00	g	140	4.0	28.6	220.00	74.10	72.40	1.00
	1.00	pc							
muffins, english, whole wheat	100.00	g	203	8.8	40.4	364.00	210.0	282.0	2.10
	66.00	g	134	5.8	26.7	240.00	139.0	186.0	1.39
	1.00	pc							

BREADS

BREADS	SERVING QUANTITY	SERVING UNIT	CALORIES (kCal)	PROTEIN (g)	TOTAL CARBOHYDRATES (g)	SODIUM (mg)	POTASSIUM (mg)	PHOSPHORUS (mg)	TOTAL FAT (g)
muffins, english,	100.00	g	235	9.1	46.3	298.00	156.0	81.00	1.80
mixed-grain includes granola	66.00	g	155	6.0	30.6	197.00	103.0	53.40	1.19
	1.00	pc							
pumpernickle,	100.00	g	250	8.7	47.5	596.00	208.0	178.0	3.10
med or regular slice	32.00	g	80	2.8	15.2	191.00	66.60	57.00	0.99
	1.00	pc							
cinammon, medium or regular slice	100.00	g	253	7.1	44.4	388.00	74.00	57.00	5.29
	28.00	g	71	2.0	12.4	109.00	20.70	16.00	1.48
	1.00	pc							
raisin, med or regular slice	100.00	g	273	8.8	52.2	432.00	180.0	112.0	3.26
	28.00	g	76	2.5	14.6	121.00	50.40	31.40	0.91
	1.00	pc							
roll, multigrain med, reg, sandwich size	100.00	g	263	9.6	44.6	458.00	160.0	122.0	6.00
	43.00	g	113	4.1	19.2	197.00	68.80	52.50	2.58
	1.00	pc							
bread stuffing, homemade	100.00	g	177	3.1	21.7	471.00	72.00	41.00	8.51
dry mix, prepared	228.00	g	404	7.2	49.5	1,070	164.0	93.50	19.40
	1.00	pc							

GRITS

GRITS	SERVING QUANTITY	SERVING UNIT	CALORIES (kCal)	PROTEIN (g)	TOTAL CARBOHYDRATES (g)	SODIUM (mg)	POTASSIUM (mg)	PHOSPHORUS (mg)	TOTAL FAT (g)
corn, yellow,	100.00	g	59	1.4	12.9	2.00	21.00	11.00	0.19
quick, unenriched	242.00	g	143	3.4	31.2	4.84	50.82	26.62	0.46
cooked with water, no salt	1.00	c							
corn, white,	100.00	g	59	1.4	12.9	2.00	21.00	11.00	0.19
quick, unenriched	242.00	g	143	3.4	31.2	4.84	50.82	26.62	0.46
cooked with water	1.00	c							
POLENTA	100.00	g							
(cornmeal)	240.00	g	139	2.7	30.	170.00	50.40	36.00	0.67
	1	c							

PASTA

	SERVING QUANTITY	SERVING UNIT	CALORIES (kcal)	PROTEIN (g)	TOTAL CARBOHYDRATES (g)	SODIUM (mg)	POTASSIUM (mg)	PHOSPHORUS (mg)	TOTAL FAT (g)
spaghetti, unenriched, cooked	100.00	g	158	5.8	30.9	1.00	44.00	58.00	0.93
	70.00	g	111	4.1	21.6	0.70	30.80	40.60	0.65
	0.50	c							
spaghetti, enriched, cooked	100.00	g	158	5.8	30.9	1.00	44.00	58.00	0.93
	140.00	g	221	8.1	43.2	1.40	61.60	81.20	1.30
	1.00	c							
spaghetti, whole wheat, cooked	100.00	g	149	6.0	30.1	4.00	96.00	127.0	1.71
	140.00	g	209	8.4	42.1	5.60	134.4	177.8	2.39
	1.00	c							
bowtie/farfalle, enriched, cooked	100.00	g	136	4.8	27.4	1.10	24.51	-na-	0.55
	154.79	g	210	7.4	42.3	0.16	37.93	-na-	0.86
	1.00	c							
fusilli, enriched, cooked	100.00	g	161	5.7	32.5	1.30	29.09	-na-	0.66
	130.41	g	210	7.4	42.3	1.70	37.93	-na-	0.86
	1.00	c							
penne, enriched, cooked	100.00	g	169	6.0	34.1	1.37	30.55	-na-	0.69
	124.17	g	210	7.4	42.3	1.70	37.93	-na-	0.86
	1.00	c							
macaroni, enriched, cooked	100.00	g	133	4.7	26.8	1.08	24.04	-na-	0.54
	157.79	g	210	7.4	42.3	1.70	37.93	-na-	0.86
	1.00	c							
lasagna, enriched, boiled/drained	100.00	g	150	5.3	30.1	1.21	26.98	-na-	0.61
	140.62	g	210	7.4	42.3	1.70	37.93	-na-	0.86
	1.00	c							
whole grain, 51%whole wheat rest enriched semolina, cooked spaghetti, unenriched, cooked	100.00	g	156	5.7	30.9	4.00	71.00	97.00	1.48

CRACKERS	SERVING QUANTITY	SERVING UNIT	CALORIES (kcal)	PROTEIN (g)	TOTAL CARBOHYDRATES (g)	SODIUM (mg)	POTASSIUM (mg)	PHOSPHORUS (mg)	TOTAL FAT (g)
melba toast, rye 3 3/4" x 1 3/4" x 1/8"	100.00	g	389	11.6	77.3	899.00	193.0	183.0	3.40
	15.00	g	58	1.7	11.6	134.85	28.95	27.45	0.51
	3.00	pcs							
melba toast, wheat	100.00	g	374	12.9	76.4	837.00	148.0	165.0	2.30
	15.00	g	56	1.9	11.5	125.55	22.20	24.75	0.35
	3.00	pcs							
saltine, low salt (square)	100.00	g	421	9.5	74.3	198.00	724.0	111.0	8.85
	15.00	g	63	1.4	11.2	29.70	108.6	16.65	1.33
	5.00	pcs							
saltine, fat-free, low sodium	100.00	g	393	10.5	82.3	849.00	115.0	113.0	1.60
	15.00	g	59	1.6	12.4	127.35	17.25	16.95	0.24
	3.00	pcs							
saltines, whole wheat/multi-grain	100.00	g	398	7.1	68.3	1,214	221.0	196.0	10.71
	14.00	g	56	1.0	9.6	169.96	30.94	27.44	1.50
	1.00	svg							
whole wheat, low salt	100.00	g	443	8.8	68.6	186.00	297.0	295.0	17.20
	28.00	g	124	2.5	19.2	52.08	83.16	82.60	4.82
	7.00	pcs							
whole wheat, reduced fat 1 svg= 29g	100.00	g	416	11.3	75.5	745.00	373.0	364.0	7.59
	4.20	g	17	0.5	3.2	31.29	15.67	15.29	0.32
	1.00	pcs							
graham, plain or honey, low fat	100.00	g	386	5.7	78.0	629.00	171.0	163.0	5.71
	35.00	g	135	2.0	27.3	220.15	59.85	57.05	2.00
	1.00	svg							
goldfish (fish-shaped), flavored	100.00	g	463	10.2	65.7	970.00	224.0	167.0	17.71
	5.20	g	24	0.5	3.4	50.44	11.65	8.68	0.92
	10.00	pcs							
toast thins, low sodium	100.00	g	442	6.5	67.7	177.00	306.0	266.0	16.13
	31.00	g	137	2.0	21.0	54.87	94.86	82.46	5.00
	1.00	svg							

Conclusion

Living with Chronic Kidney Disease (CKD) is a long-term journey. It requires resilience, patience, and a willingness to stay informed. The purpose of this guide has always been simple: to give you the knowledge and tools needed to take an active role in your kidney health.

Understanding CKD, its causes, symptoms, and progression - is the first step. When you understand what's happening inside your body, you're no longer navigating in the dark. Regular monitoring and consistent follow-up with your healthcare team help you make informed decisions and adjust your plan as needed.

Nutrition remains one of the most powerful tools available to you. Managing potassium, phosphorus, sodium, protein, and fluids can feel detailed at times, but each thoughtful choice matters. The food lists and meal planning guidance in this book are designed to help you build meals with clarity and confidence.

Managing CKD requires **consistency**. Small, steady improvements in your daily habits can create meaningful change over time. With the right structure and knowledge, you can move forward feeling informed, prepared, and supported.

Meal Planning

Your diet is the foundation of managing CKD. While shifting to a renal-friendly way of eating might appear overwhelming at first, by following a clear structure, meal planning becomes far more manageable.

The food lists in this guide are meant to be your daily roadmap. By understanding how to balance potassium, phosphorus, sodium, and protein, along with your fluid intake, you can build meals that support your specific stage of CKD with confidence.

This isn't just about avoiding certain foods; rather, it's about discovering kidney-friendly options that protect your health while still allowing you to enjoy what you eat.

Portion Control and Nutrition Labels

Mastering your environment is just as important as knowing what to eat. The grocery store doesn't have to be a source of stress. Armed with the skills to decode nutrition labels and a strong grasp of portion control, you can shop and prepare food with confidence.

Rely on the practical grocery tips and the diverse recipe sections (covering breakfast, lunch, dinner, snacks, and beverages) to keep your meals varied. These tools ensure your daily routine remains satisfying and enjoyable while keeping your lab results on track.

Knowledge is Power

Living with CKD also involves dispelling myths and understanding the facts about the condition. Knowledge is empowering and can help you take control of your health.

Coping strategies and effective collaboration with your healthcare providers are integral to managing CKD. Open communication with your healthcare team can significantly enhance the effectiveness of your care.

Final Thoughts

While CKD may necessitate specific lifestyle adjustments, having a well-researched food list at your disposal empowers you to take charge of your health. As you implement these changes, be sure to work closely with your doctor and healthcare team to regularly monitor your labs and ensure your new habits are keeping you on track.

Every positive choice you make at the dinner table is a victory for your well-being. You are not alone on this journey. Take it one meal and one day at a time. With the right knowledge and support, you can successfully manage CKD and continue living a happy, fulfilling life.

Appendix A: Glossary

A

- Albumin: A protein in the blood that can indicate kidney function when found in urine.

- Albuminuria: A condition characterized by an excessive amount of the protein albumin in the urine, often indicating kidney damage.

B

- Blood Levels: A term referring to the amount of a particular substance, such as potassium or phosphorus, present in the blood.

- Body Weight: A person's mass or weight, typically measured in kilograms.

C

- Caloric Intake: The total amount of calories consumed in a day, which can vary based on factors like age, sex, weight, and physical activity level.

- Calories: A unit used to measure the amount of energy that food provides when eaten and digested.

- Carbohydrates: One of the three macronutrients, along with protein and fat; carbohydrates are important sources of energy for the body.

- Chronic Kidney Disease (CKD): A long-term condition where the kidneys do not work as well as normal, leading to progressive loss of kidney function.

- Dietary Fiber: Nutrient in our diet that is not digested by gastrointestinal enzymes but fulfills an important role for digestive health.

- Dietitian: A healthcare professional who specializes in diet and nutrition, providing personalized dietary advice based on specific needs and health conditions.

- Dietary Guidelines: Recommendations provided by reputable scientific organizations pertaining to health and nutrition.

D

- Dialysis: A treatment that filters and purifies the blood using a machine to maintain balance in the body when the kidneys cannot perform these functions.

- Diabetes: A chronic disease affecting the body's ability to use sugar for energy, potentially leading to high blood sugar levels and kidney damage.

- Dietary Requirements: The levels of intake of essential nutrients considered adequate to meet the known nutritional needs of practically all healthy people.

E

- End-Stage Renal Disease (ESRD): A term used when kidney failure reaches an advanced stage, necessitating dialysis or kidney transplantation.

F

- Fats: One of the three main macronutrients, along with carbohydrates and protein; fats are a concentrated source of energy.

- Glomerular Filtration Rate (GFR): A test used to assess how well the kidneys are functioning, specifically estimating how much blood passes through the glomeruli each minute.

H

- Hemodialysis: A treatment for kidney failure that uses a machine to filter the patient's blood outside the body and return it back to circulation.

- Healthcare Provider: A person who helps prevent or treat illness or injury, including doctors, nurses, and allied health professionals.

- Hypertension: Also known as high blood pressure, a condition that can damage blood vessels and organs, including the kidneys.

K

- Kidney Failure: A condition in which the kidneys lose their ability to function properly, often requiring dialysis or transplantation.

- Kidney Function: The ability of the kidneys to filter waste products from the blood and regulate fluid and electrolyte balance.

- Kilogram: The basic unit of mass in the metric system, commonly used to measure body weight.

- Potassium: An essential nutrient that helps nerves and muscles communicate and assists in moving nutrients into cells and waste products out of cells. Excess potassium can be harmful in CKD.

M

- Management: The process of dealing with or controlling health conditions, particularly in the context of chronic illnesses like CKD.

- Myths: Common misconceptions or false beliefs about a subject, such as chronic kidney disease.

N

- Nephrologist: A doctor who specializes in diagnosing and treating diseases of the kidneys.

- Nutrient Requirements: The levels of intake of essential nutrients considered adequate to meet the known nutritional needs of practically all healthy people.

- Peritoneal Dialysis: A treatment for patients with severe chronic kidney disease where sterile fluid containing glucose is introduced into the abdomen, absorbs waste products, and is then drained out.

P

- Phosphorus: A mineral crucial for healthy bones and teeth; excess phosphorus levels can indicate impaired kidney function.

- Physical Activity Level: A measure of a person's daily physical activity, used to estimate total energy expenditure.

- Portion Control: The practice of managing the amount of food consumed in one sitting, which can help control calorie intake.

- Protein: A macronutrient essential for building muscle mass and overall health; its intake may need to be monitored in CKD.

- Proteinuria: The presence of excess proteins in the urine, often indicative of kidney damage.

- Renal Dietitian: A dietitian who specializes in the dietary management of diseases affecting the kidneys, providing personalized advice to patients with CKD.

S

- Serving Size: The amount of food or drink that is generally served, used to quantify recommended amounts, nutrient content, and caloric values in dietary guidelines and food labels.

- Sodium: A mineral crucial for maintaining blood pressure and fluid balance; CKD patients may have difficulty regulating sodium levels.

- Trans Fat: A type of dietary fat associated with an increased risk of heart disease.

- Unsaturated Fats: Healthy fats that are liquid at room temperature, such as olive oil and canola oil, which can help improve cholesterol levels.

U

- Uremia: A high level of waste products in the blood due to poor kidney function or kidney failure.

- Urine: Liquid waste produced by the kidneys and excreted by the body; in CKD, the kidneys may not effectively produce urine.

V

- Vitamins: Organic compounds required by the body in small amounts to sustain life; essential for various bodily functions.

- World Health Organization (WHO): A specialized agency of the United Nations responsible for international public health.

Appendix B: Resources

BIDMC Food Prioritization Project by https://www.renaltracker.com
Food List Reference: USDA FoodData Central – https://www.fdc.nal.usda.gov

The Basics of a Kidney-Friendly Diet:
1. National Kidney Foundation. (2015). A to Z Health Guide. https://www.kidney.org/atoz/content/diet
2. Kidney Care UK. (2021). Fluid control for kidney patients. https://www.kidneycareuk.org/about-kidney-health/living-kidney-disease/kidney-kitchen/factsheets/fluid-control-kidney-patients/
3. National Institute of Diabetes and Digestive and Kidney Diseases. (2017). Eating & Nutrition for Hemodialysis. https://www.niddk.nih.gov/health-information/kidney-disease/kidney-failure/hemodialysis/eating-nutrition

Meal Planning for Kidney Health
1. National Kidney Foundation: Nutrition and Chronic Kidney Disease (Stages 1–4) https://www.kidney.org/atoz/content/nutrichronic
2. National Kidney Foundation: Nutrition and Early Kidney Disease (Stages 1–4)
   https://www.kidney.org/sites/default/files/11-50-0113_patbro_nutrition.pdf
3. National Kidney Foundation: Potassium and Your CKD Diet
   https://www.kidney.org/atoz/content/potassium
4. National Kidney Foundation: Phosphorus and Your CKD Diet
   https://www.kidney.org/atoz/content/phosphorus
5. American Dietetic Association: Chronic Kidney Disease (CKD) and Diet: Assessment, Management, and Treatment
   https://www.eatrightpro.org/-/media/eatrightpro-files/practice/position-and-practice-papers/position-papers/kidneydisease.pdf
6. World Health Organization: Protein and Amino Acid Requirements in Human Nutrition
   https://www.who.int/nutrition/publications/nutrientrequirements/WHO_TRS_935/en/
7. Dietary Guidelines for Americans
   https://www.dietaryguidelines.gov/sites/default/files/2019-05/2015-2020_Dietary_Guidelines.pdf

Portion Control and Serving Sizes
1. https://www.niddk.nih.gov/health-information/weight-management/just-enough-food-portions
2. Food Portioning: www.covenanthome.care

Myths and Facts about CKD
1. National Kidney Foundation: 10 Common Myths About Chronic Kidney Disease
   https://www.kidney.org/news/ekidney/march_2013/myths
2. American Kidney Fund: Kidney disease facts
   https://www.kidneyfund.org/kidney-disease/kidney-disease-facts/
3. National Institute of Diabetes and Digestive and Kidney Diseases: Eating & Nutrition for Hemodialysis
   https://www.niddk.nih.gov/health-information/kidney-disease/kidney-failure/hemodialysis/eating-nutrition
4. Mayo Clinic: Chronic kidney disease
   https://www.mayoclinic.org/diseases-conditions/chronic-kidney-disease/symptoms-causes/syc-20354521

Appendix C: Index

www.ingramcontent.com/pod-product-compliance
Lightning Source LLC
Chambersburg PA
CBHW060228030426
42335CB00014B/1374